Productivity at the Workstation

Maintaining Fitness at Your Desk

Robert Regis Dvorak

CRISP PUBLICATIONS, INC.
Los Altos, California

Productivity
at the Workstation
Maintaining Fitness at Your Desk

Robert Regis Dvorak

CREDITS
Editor: **Anne Knight**
Design and Composition: **Interface Studio**
Cover Design: **Carol Harris**
Illustration: **Robert Regis Dvorak**

Copyright © 1990 by Robert Regis Dvorak
Printed in the United States of America

Crisp books are distributed in Canada by Reid Publishing, Ltd., P.O. Box 7267, Oakville, Ontario, Canada L6J 6L6.

In Australia by Career Builders, P.O. Box 1051, Springwood, Brisbane, Queensland, Australia 4127.

And in New Zealand by Career Builders, P.O. Box 571, Manurewa, New Zealand.

Library of Congress Catalog Card Number 89-82344
Dvorak, Robert R.
Productivity at the Workstation
ISBN 1-56052-041-8

PREFACE

Why do we need a book titled *Productivity at the Workstation*? What's the big deal? Just sit down and do your job. Got a problem? Hang in there. Probably no one ever told you that sitting at a computer workstation can be hazardous to your health—but then so can driving a car and walking across the street. Let's set things straight! A person invented the chair. And, as usual, when humans invent something there can be mistaken assumptions and miscalculations. Humans also invented the visual display terminal (VDT). Put the two together in a workplace designed for typewriters, and you have problems in Computer City.

This book has been written primarily for you if you are a worker whose job it is to spend hours sitting at a desk or workstation with a typewriter or VDT and keyboard. Its purpose is to help you create a program to help you be more productive and feel great at the same time.

I have included many suggestions for exercise, movement, diet, sleep, posture, work habits, vision care, and mental balance. Many are new and will not be found in any other book. Others you undoubtedly have heard or seen before. Owing to the inactive sedentary work station routine, I feel compelled to emphasize their importance. A well-maintained body is free from symptoms of backaches, muscle tension, stiff neck, eye strain, headaches, numbness, nerve problems, and other disorders frequently experienced as a result of sitting at a desk for long periods of time. This book is designed to make you aware of your environment and teach you how to care for your body so that you can work with greater comfort and productivity. This is not a medical program but an educational one. If you have persistent health problems, the supervision of a qualified health care professional is recommended.

When the suggestions in the book are followed, you can expect greater comfort, more energy, enhanced performance, and higher productivity. When employees are happier and less stressed, productivity increases and absenteeism declines. Employee fitness and well-being promote optimum mental performance, which are essential for productive, error-free work.

Productivity at the Workstation will assist you in assessing your workstation and your own body. It will help you to identify your problem areas and adjust your workspace and its tools to fit and accommodate your needs. This is called "ergonomics."

i

As you proceed through this book, you are likely to realize a new awareness of yourself and your environment. I believe that awareness is the most important lesson to be learned. With increased awareness, you will naturally and willingly assume greater control over your work environment and your body. Most of the suggestions are ones that I practice myself and find work well for me. But don't expect to change all your habits overnight. I didn't.

Most of us *know* what is best for ourselves intuitively, but we don't always consistently *do* what is best. This book can assist you in staying on target. Begin with what you feel is your top priority. And the most important advice I can give is *begin!* Make the commitment to initiate your program *now* to make the changes necessary to enhance your comfort and performance at the workstation.

Robert Regis Dvorak

CONTENTS

Preface i

PART I **INTRODUCTION** 1
What is Fitness? 2
How This Book Can Help You 4

PART II **ASSESSMENT OF YOUR PHYSICAL CONDITION** 7
How Do You Feel Right Now? 8
Stress 10
"Type A" Behavior 12
Immobility 13
Full-Spectrum Lighting 14
Posture 16
Diet 18

PART III **INITIATING AND MAINTAINING NEW HABITS** 21
The Office Environment 22
Your Workstation 29
Your Body 44
Your Habits 46
Fitness at the Desk 48
   Sitting 48
   Standing 53
   Rest and Relaxation 54
   Breathing for Life 56
   Wrists, Hands and Fingers 57
   Leg and Foot Care 61
   Stretching 62
   Exercise 65
   Movement Exercises for People Who Sit at Work 67
   Posture Perfect 71
   Massage 73
   Eating and Drinking 75
   Diet and Food Recommendations 76
   The Hurry Habit 78
   The Mini-Break 80
   Psychological Pressure 81
   Sleep 82

(Contents continued next page)

CONTENTS (Continued)

PART IV VISION CARE..85
    Your Eyes: A Barometer of Health 86
    How Eyes Work..87
    Causes of Eyestrain and Tension 89
    How to Minimize Eyestrain and Tension at the Workstation 92

PART V DEVELOPING A PERSONAL ACTION PLAN 94
    Goal Setting 95
    Recommendations In Brief.....................................96
    Suggested readings 97

PART I

INTRODUCTION

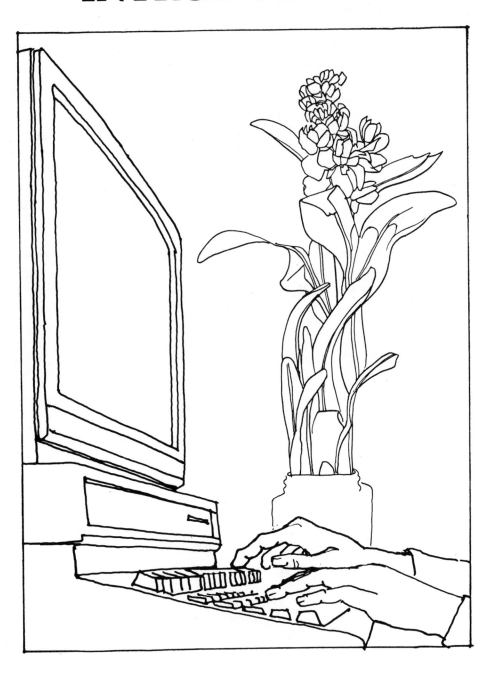

WHAT IS FITNESS?

In the abridged version of *Webster's New World Dictionary*, the third verb definition of "fit" is "to adjust so as to fit." The third adjective definition of "fit" is "healthy." That says it. The following pages will help you adjust to fit your situation of sitting down at a desk to do your work every work day. Traditionally, we have considered desk jobs "soft jobs." But we now know that it is very hard on our bodies to sit all day. It requires a real effort to develop those habits that will keep us vibrantly alive while in a sitting posture.

People who work at a desk and are not fit can lack the motivation to be productive and assume the job's responsibilities. They may also experience body pain, eye strain, headaches, backaches, and other physical discomforts. They may feel tired and lethargic. They may drink a lot of coffee to get through the day. They may even resort to other drugs. For an unfit person, work will not be much fun, and he or she will derive little satisfaction other than a pay check. The employee loses and so does the employer. Unfortunately, this state of affairs is far too common.

Fitness at the workstation means feeling mentally and physically vibrant, healthy, energetic, and happy. It means being free of physical pain and dependence on drugs, alcohol, or any other harmful substances—even excessive use of coffee and sugar. It means having the energy to handle whatever your job requires. When you are fit, you enjoy the challenges and the opportunities your job offers. Your work is more than a job: it is a place to learn and grow. When you are fit, you feel in control of yourself and your environment. Your employer benefits and so do you.

A WORD OF CAUTION

When you heed the suggestions in this book and perform the exercises, you will be changing habits and your working environment, decreasing your discomfort, and increasing your productivity and pleasure. You know your present limitations. Change and growth take time. Proceed with caution and at your own pace. If you are now under the care of a physician, chiropractor, or ophthalmologist, be sure to get medical approval before embarking on this guided journey. Listen to what your body tells you. Become aware of how you are feeling day by day and minute by minute. Be aware that sometimes physical changes can make you ache, sore, or stiff. This is normal. But if you have any medical questions or concerns, consult a qualified professional.

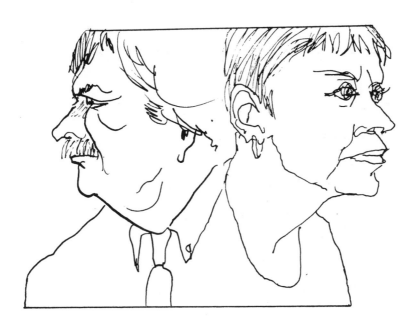

HOW THIS BOOK CAN HELP YOU: WHAT'S THE PAY-OFF?

In order to change a habit or a way of doing something, it is first necessary to have a reason for doing so. The more reasons we have to change something, the more motivated we will be to accomplish our goal. The two main motivations for doing anything are:

1. Eliminating pain
2. Experiencing pleasure

Write below all of the benefits you can think of for initiating change. Ask yourself, "How would I like my life and work to be different? If it could be the very best, what would it be like? What are the pay-offs?" Get a clear picture in your mind of what your ideal situation could be.

BENEFIT LIST

Here are some benefits for starters. Check those that apply to you.

_____ I will feel much better than I do now.

_____ I will feel more in control of my working environment.

_____ I will like my body better.

_____ I will stay younger longer.

_____ I will have more energy.

_____ I will have a better attendance record.

_____ I will feel vibrantly alive.

_____ I will experience less pain.

_____ My eyes will be stronger.

_____ I will have little or no eye strain.

_____ The chronic tension in my neck and shoulders will be gone.

_____ I will not experience headaches due to eye tension.

_____ I will be happier.

_____ I will be more efficient.

_____ I will feel more physically comfortable.

_____ I will be less stressed.

_____ I will feel more positive, and this will reflect on my fellow workers.

_____ I will have more satisfaction, because I will get my work done faster.

_____ I won't feel tired at work any more.

_____ I will have a strong, positive attitude about my work.

_____ I will be able to get along better with the others at my job.

_____ I will have more fun on the job.

_____ I will enjoy the challenges of work.

_____ My increased job performance will yield me a much higher income.

_____ I will no longer be dependent on drugs, alcohol, or stimulants.

_____ I will be able to concentrate again.

_____ I will not be so dependent on my glasses.

_____ I will enjoy going to work.

_____ I will feel better during my nonworking hours.

_____ I will have more friends.

_____ I will be able to help others be more productive and feel better.

Add your own: _____

_____

_____

_____

_____

_____

_____

_____

PART II

ASSESSMENT OF YOUR PHYSICAL CONDITION

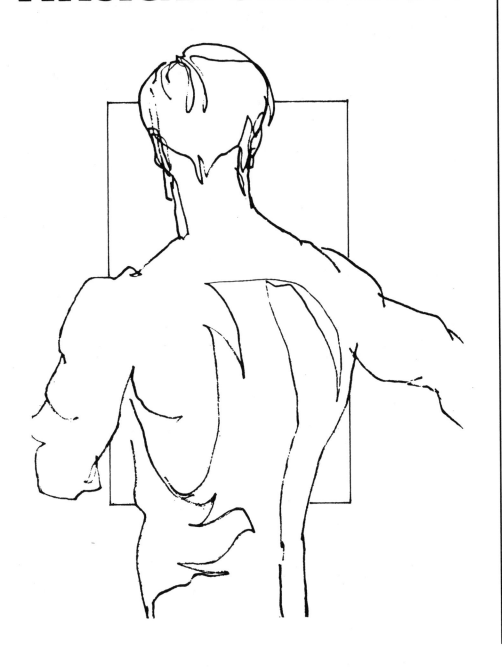

HOW DO YOU FEEL RIGHT NOW?

Make a survey of your physical comfort. Discover what needs to be improved. Which of these two statements apply to you?

_____ I am currently experiencing discomfort.

_____ I sometimes experience discomfort.

Now identify your discomfort and locate where it occurs. Check what applies to you:

___ Body fatigue	___ Backache	___ Pain in the wrists
___ Neck tension	___ Neck pain	___ Digestive problems
___ Burning eyes	___ Vision loss	___ Eye strain
___ Blurry vision	___ Leg cramps	___ Shoulder pain
___ Dry eyes	___ Headaches	___ Light-sensitive eyes
___ Wrist strain	___ Overweight	___ Underweight
___ Dry skin	___ Impulsive eating	___ Swollen feet or ankles
___ Cold feet	___ Numbness	___ Arthritis in the hands
___ Nerve pain	___ Stiff neck	___ Carpal tunnel syndrome

Now, add any areas of discomfort that have not been listed:

_____   _____   _____

_____   _____   _____

_____   _____   _____

_____   _____   _____

_____   _____   _____

Now, assess how you feel about yourself and your job. Check that which applies to your situation:

___ I am not in control of my working environment.

___ I don't like my manager.

___ I don't like my body.

___ I am looking older.

___ I don't have enough energy.

___ I have a poor attendance record.

___ I feel tired at certain times during the day.

___ My eyes are getting weaker.

___ I have chronic tension in my neck and shoulders.

___ I experience headaches due to eye tension.

___ I am not happy at my desk.

___ I am not as efficient as I would like to be.

___ I tend to be forgetful.

___ I am not comfortable at my desk.

___ I don't get my work done fast enough.

___ I feel tired at work.

___ I have a negative attitude about work.

___ I'm irritable and don't get along well with the others at work.

___ Work is not fun.

___ I have a hard time meeting the challenges of work.

___ I haven't had a substantial raise in two years.

___ I depend on drugs, alcohol, or stimulants.

___ I have trouble concentrating.

___ I am dependent on my glasses.

___ I don't enjoy going to work.

___ When I'm off work, I lack the energy to do much.

___ I have a cynical or negative attitude.

If you checked three or fewer statements, you are doing great. But if you checked more than three you have some work to do. The more you checked the more you need to initiate a program similar to the one described in this book.

STRESS

Many factors contribute to physical and mental fatigue, pain, and other discomfort. Simply being alive stresses the mind and body. A certain amount of stress is necessary to keep the body strong, healthy, and in condition. A weight lifter intentionally stresses his or her muscles to build strength. Stress is natural, inevitable, and it can be beneficial. It is what we do with it or how we work with it that can be a problem. The body is amazing. Not only do we cope with the inevitable daily stresses, but we add other stresses that weaken this amazing system. Some people eat poorly, smoke, drink alcohol in excess, take drugs that alter body chemistry, slouch, eat excessive amounts of sugar, are overweight, don't get enough sleep, work too much, etc. The body is wonderful, because it lets us know when we are treating it badly. We feel weaker, get sick, have frequent colds, ache, have muscle pains, and look older when we have poor health habits. Eliminating these poor habits can give your amazing system new life, energy, and vitality.

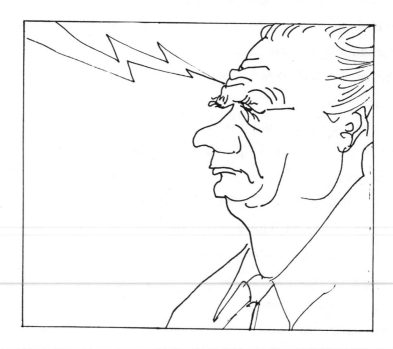

MENTAL STRESS

Where is your mind? In your head? In your brain?

I like to think of the mind as being located *everywhere* in the body. In fact, for most purposes you can consider the mind as your body. There is no separation. Even if you think of your mind as your brain, you will have to admit that all the parts of your body are connected to it by way of the nervous system. The mind is responsible for keeping every part of the body in good working order.

It is very important how you talk to yourself about your body. If you get up in the morning with the attitude that you are still tired or that you feel awful, your mind will help fulfill that idea for you. Be careful what you say to yourself. The mind does what we tell it to do. Exercise your mind power and keep it fresh and alert by encouraging creativity and vitality throughout your day. For the next week, write down any negative thought patterns that you recognize need changing. Catch yourself saying to yourself—or out loud—such phrases as:

> I'm tired.
> I'm sick and tired.
> This work is a pain in the neck.
> What a pain!
> Oh, my aching back.
> He (or she) makes me sick.
> My boss, this job, is a pain in the neck.

Every time you catch yourself making one of these comments, write it here:

_____

_____

_____

_____

_____

_____

_____

"TYPE A" BEHAVIOR

"Type A" behavior as described by researchers Friedman and Sosenman is the overstressed life style that can result in a heart attack. Type A behavior is characterized by what some call the "hurry and worry habit."

You can tell if you are a Type A personality if you are:

(Check the box that applies)

	Often	Sometimes	Never
Impatient with others at work.	☐	☐	☐
Feel the world is going too slow for you.	☐	☐	☐
Think that you succeed because you do your job faster than others.	☐	☐	☐
Move, talk, eat, and walk fast.	☐	☐	☐
Become irritated or even angry at slower drivers on the road.	☐	☐	☐
Become angry because you didn't get enough work done in a day.	☐	☐	☐
Are forever playing catch up.	☐	☐	☐
Become irritated when others are late for appointments.	☐	☐	☐
Are often late for appointments yourself because you try to squeeze just one last short task in before leaving.	☐	☐	☐
Criticize yourself or others when a time-wasting mistake is made.	☐	☐	☐
Misplace your keys or glasses.	☐	☐	☐

Most Type A symptoms are a result of not operating in present time and being unaware of the pleasure of living moment by moment. The Type A personality lives in past (with regrets) or future (with expectations) time awareness. The fact is that the real enjoyment of life is lost in self-imposed worry and time pressure.

IMMOBILITY

Life is movement. Everythng that lives is in motion. The earth turns, the heart
beats, and the blood circulates. Movement is life. However, a job sitting at a
workstation or desk is characterized by immobility. Fingers and hands move, the
head moves, but that is about it. Immobility is one of the main causes of body
tightness, muscle pain, cramps, stiff neck, backache, etc. Immobility also
underlies many vision problems, which can result in headaches, poorer eyesight,
burning eyes, and eye strain. Anything you can do to increase mobility at your
workstation will make you feel better. Later in this book you will be given specific
suggestions for maximizing mobility.

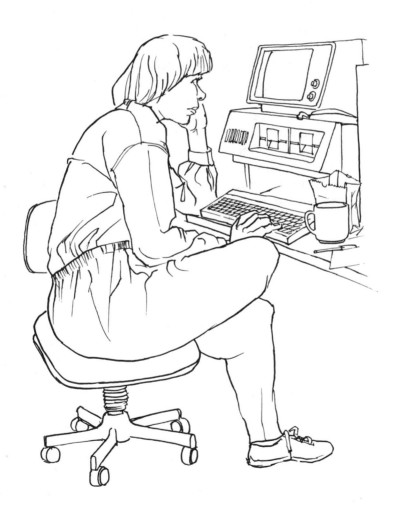

FULL-SPECTRUM LIGHTING

Sunlight rates along with food, air, and water as essential to the survival of human life on our planet. Solar radiation activates primary biochemical events in the body which influence our biological clocks, circadian rhythms, immunologic response, sexual activity, regulation of stress, control of viral infections, and strength of the nervous system.

We do not yet know the full effect of artificial light on living systems. Studies have shown, however, that the wrong kind of artificial lighting can make workers irritable, sluggish, and reduce productivity. Researchers agree that light is essential to life and is required for the full functioning of the endocrine system. The wrong kind of lighting interferes with calcium absorption, contributing to brittle bones in older people. Photobiologists, scientists specializing in the study of lighting effects on humans and animals, say that most incandescent bulbs and most fluorescent bulbs do not produce full-spectrum light—light that approximates our sun's color-balancing wavelengths.

Certainly there are many benefits from exposure to full-spectrum light. Scientific studies in the Soviet Union have shown that under full-spectrum light, production goes up and absenteeism goes down. Now many Soviet workplaces mandate this type of light. The Soviets also offer ''light therapy'' for coal miners. This treatment requires miners to disrobe and spend one-half hour each day in natural or full-spectrum artificial lighting. This practice has been useful both in preventing and in treating black lung disease. Soviet studies have also shown that full-spectrum light gives the body an increased tolerance to environmental pollution.

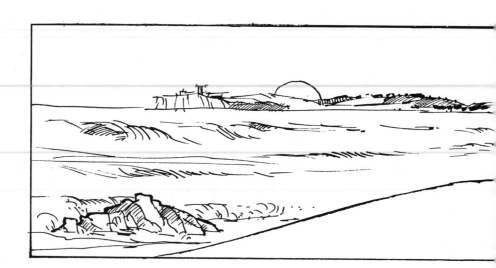

The beneficial effect of full-spectrum light is well known in the dairy industry and the horticulture industry. Full-spectrum light has medical and psychological applications. It has been used to treat psoriasis, neonatal jaundice, and herpes simplex infections. Studies conducted in schools have shown that full-spectrum lighting improves academic performance, children's behavior, and reduces fatigue.

How does full-spectrum light work to benefit us? Natural sunlight stimulates the pineal gland, a pea-sized organ in the head. This gland secretes melatonin, a hormone that seems to control many bodily functions. Both plastic and glass eyeglasses and contact lenses block some of the light rays that travel through the eye to the pineal gland. Sunlight is our chief source of Vitamin D, which is synthesized by ultraviolet light on the skin. Vitamin D promotes bone development and prevents rickets. It is even suspected that full-spectrum lighting is helpful to people suffering from arthritis.

In the 1970's, in experiments with first graders in Sarasota, Florida, researchers found that children who were working in a classroom with cool, white fluorescent lighting were much more hyperactive than students in another classroom where full-spectrum tubes duplicated natural sunlight but had shields filtering out harmful radiation. Under the cool white fluorescents, students exhibited nervous fatigue, irritability, lapses of attention, and hyperactive behavior.

In a Cornell University study at the Center for Improvement of Undergraduate Education, students working under full-spectrum fluorescent lighting experienced a significant increase in visual acuity and a reduction in overall fatigue compared to their performance under regular fluorescent lights.

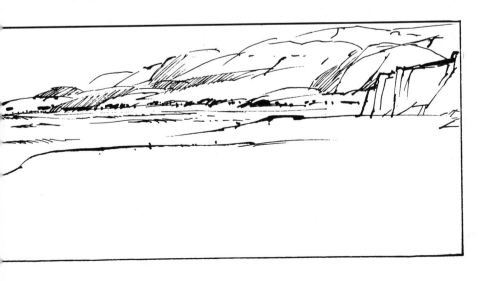

POSTURE

"Think posture perfect."

When we sit or stand with perfect posture, we maintain the natural curvature of our spine, and our bodies are balanced and relaxed. It sounds easy. Why then, does it feel so good to slouch or slump in our chairs at times? Slumping usually occurs when the muscles get tired holding a certain posture for long periods of time without movement. It is the body's attempt to take the strain and tension away from these muscles.

The attempt to relieve strained muscles by slumping requires greater muscular effort, increases body tension, and burdens the spine by creating pressure on the discs between the vertebrae.

The force of gravity is constantly "pulling" us toward the ground. When we keep our body aligned and in balance, gravity helps to keep us that way. The more balanced we are, the less energy it takes to stand or sit.

Many people say that they get tired when maintaining good posture, but it is their *habit* of poor posture, sometimes resulting from years of holding the body unnaturally, that makes good posture feel awkward. When the habitual slouch becomes the norm, correct posture is the difficult exception. When good posture is habitual, the opposite is true. Good posture is easier on our bodies because it brings our body into alignment, with less muscle tension, which in turn makes for improved health and increased productivity.

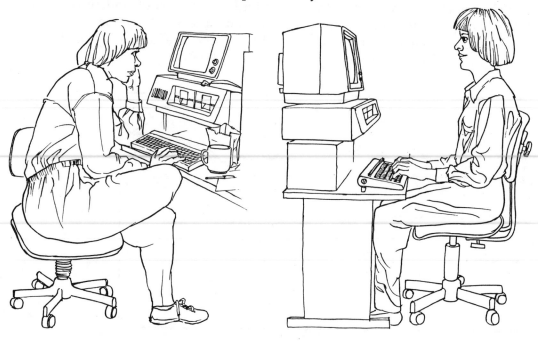

Poor posture may reflect psychological insecurity. Because posture reflects our mental set, poor self-image can result in poor posture. People who feel good about themselves stand tall, proud to be who they are. The military forces know that good posture raises morale, and requires men and women in military service to stand tall.

Posture problems can result from sitting in a chair that does not fit the body, sitting for long periods in one position, sitting or standing habits that are unbalanced, or poor muscle tone. Our muscles are meant to hold the natural S curve of the spine. When we change these curves while sitting, we can increase the pressure on the discs. This can eventually cause back pain and require professional care.

When we lean on our arms or rest our head on our hands with the elbow propped up on the desk, we put our head, neck, and shoulders into a state of immobility. Immobility tightens our muscles, causing neck and shoulder cramps, eye strain, and headaches. When we habitually sit hunched over or slouch, we cause unnecessary muscle tension and pressure on the disks between the vertebrae of the spine. We have to work harder to think and breathe, and our body requires more energy to maintain circulation. If our bad posture continues unchanged, our bodies adapt to the abnormal posture. Eventually painful problems can result. For example, when we stand and sit with our body in alignment, we feel better, breathe better, and think better.

Exercise: Get to know your posture. Rate yourself.

	Perfect	Good	Fair	Poor
Standing				
Sitting				
Posture habits				
Balance				
Your S curve				

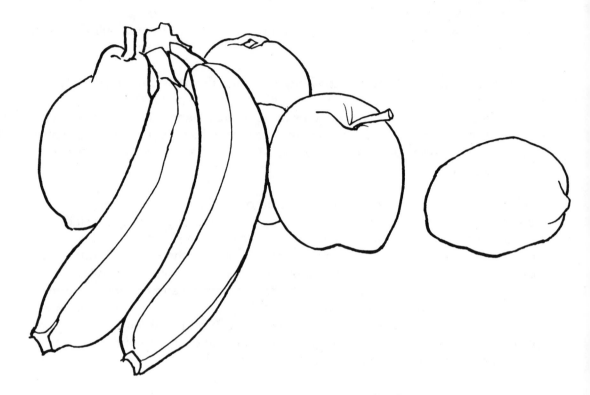

DIET

Most of us eat too much. Not just too much food, but too much wrong food such as: processed foods, rich foods, fatty foods, oily foods, preserved foods, refined sugars and starches. Improved eating habits can result in an improvement of your general health and the way you feel forever. First, become aware of what you are putting into your body each day. For one week keep a log on what you eat. Record everything that goes into your mouth. It will give you a new awareness of your eating habits and can help you change those habits. When you have completed this exercise read the material on eating and drinking on page 76, and plan an ideal week.

	BEFORE BREAKFAST	BREAKFAST	BETWEEN BREAKFAST & LUNCH	LUNCH	BETWEEN LUNCH & DINNER	DINNER	BETWEEN DINNER & SLEEP
Monday							
Tuesday							
Wednesday							
Thursday							
Friday							
Saturday							
Sunday							

PART III

INITIATING AND MAINTAINING NEW HABITS

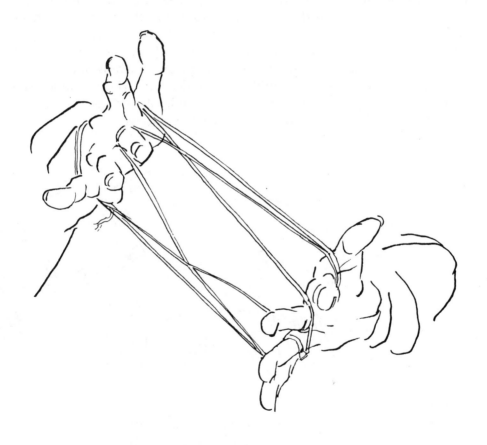

THE OFFICE ENVIRONMENT

The office environment affects your ability to work productively. Certain factors in your environment you can control, and others you can't. Take responsibility to change for the better those conditions over which you have some control. Don't be willing to put up with anything but the best possible alternatives.

Many modern, brightly lighted offices were not designed for the computer age. Those rows of fluorescent tubing overhead were designed for paper work, not for VDTs. The glare they produce on your screens makes seeing difficult. Adapting for VDT use an office that was once used for typing and hard-copy tasks requires special considerations and investment. In the office of the future, VDT workers will be able to monitor the environment and make their own adjustments. The science of ergonomics studies how people organize their environments to accommodate their kind of work. Flexibility and adaptability will be the key in bringing today's work environments into line with our electronic age. Movable, fabric-covered partitions to reduce noise and glare, movable modular furniture, controlled temperature and humidity, nonreflective surfaces, hidden cables, individual task lighting, and subdued ambient lighting all play a part in making our offices healthier and more comfortable places to work.

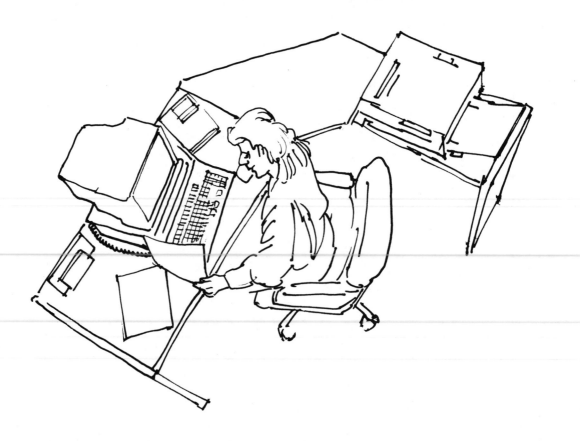

Lighting and Reflections   Most desk work involves using the eyes. Good lighting conditions are essential to productivity. Straining to see in poor light or trying to avoid reflections takes extra time and energy away from doing your job.

Any time that you have to stretch your neck, squint your eyes, or lean forward in your chair to decipher images on the screen because of poor lighting or reflections, you are giving yourself an extra workout. Squinting produces tension in your eyes; when squinting is a habit, it is very detrimental. Twisting your neck will send you to the chiropractor. Headaches and other problems can result from inadequate lighting, overbright lighting, and reflections.

Glare can be kept to a minumum by modifying light sources and the surfaces that reflect light. Shield exposed light bulbs and cover windows that produce unwanted reflections. Louvered blinds can effectively direct light away from VDT screens and still allow people to see outside. Workstation furniture and walls can have a nonreflective finish. Wearing dark clothes and avoiding sparkling jewelry will further reduce glare.

Where VDT work is the primary focus, general office lighting should be lowered. Low lighting—200 to 500 lux—is best. If you work with both VDTs and paper documents, try for a combination of low office lighting and individual task lighting—500 to 700 lux—with adjustable arm desk lamps.

THE OFFICE ENVIRONMENT (Continued)

Full-Spectrum Lighting   If your company is up-to-date, you are working under economical fluorescent lighting; see page 15 for why this kind of lighting is not the best kind for you. It is probably not prudent to try to change the system your company has installed, but it is possible to take measures of your own so that you receive adequate natural light for good health and energy. This means getting outdoors on weekends and installing full-spectrum light bulbs in your desk lamps. Full-spectrum bulbs are made by Duro-Test Corporation, North Bergen, N.H., and Lumiram Electric Corporation, Mamaroneck, New York. Don't be dissuaded by their price; they will last 100 times longer than your ordinary incandescent bulb—most are guaranteed for 4000 hours or more. Once you experience the beautiful light that they produce you will not settle for less. You will find reading is easier and that your eyes are less tired.

Temperature and Air Circulation   Maintaining the right temperature can be a problem. Ideally, you will have your own office space and can control the temperature. Most people are not so lucky. If your office is too cool for you, dress warmer and sit away from drafts. If your office is too warm, wear loose, cool clothing. It is better not to sit with a fan or blower sending warm or cool air on any part of your body. Air blowing on any part of your body, especially cool air, can make that part tighten up, causing muscle tension or misalignments of the spine, which, in turn, can pinch nerves. If you discover that you have a cool or warm air problem and can't control it yourself, get help from the office manager or facilities manager. Have a vent diverted, closed, or covered. If you can't get immediate action, take the responsibility yourself and tape cardboard over the opening until the maintenance people come to your aid. Use the blinds on windows to reduce glare and control uncomfortably warm summer temperature or seasonal cold.

Room humidity of about 50 percent is most comfortable. If you can, find out the humidity of your office. If it is low, you will have to compensate by drinking more liquids or getting a humidifer. If it is high, it affects how your body perceives the ambient temperature, making warm temperatures possibly uncomfortably warm and cool ones uncomfortably cool.

Sound If it drains your energy to filter out unwanted noise around you in order to concentrate on your work, then sound is a problem. Basically, there are two types of sound: prevailing sound and unexpected sound. The sounds that really disrupt concentration are the unpredictable noises that startle you as you work.

Examples of prevailing sounds are those produced by such machines as air conditioning fans and unintelligible conversations. Many equipment sounds can be kept to a minimum by using pads under machines and employing other types of sound insulation. Well-maintained machines are quieter than those in disrepair. If you are troubled by noise from equipment, contact the manufacturer for advice.

Distracting sounds are nearby conversations that can be understood, telephones ringing, copy machines popping out copies, footsteps, loud laughter, and anything that disrupts the norm. Telephone rings can be turned down, sound-absorbent partitions can be installed, carpeting applied to floors (and walls), and a company-wide awareness of the importance of sound courtesy can all help to reduce these distractions.

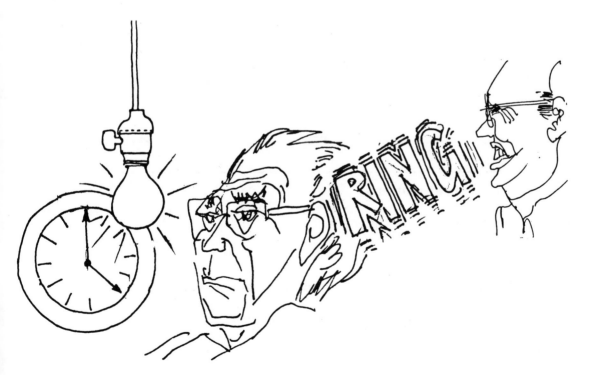

THE OFFICE ENVIRONEMNT (Continued)

Exercise Take a few minutes just to sit with your eyes closed and let yourself become aware of all the sounds that you hear. List each identifiable sound below:

_____   _____

_____   _____

_____   _____

_____   _____

_____   _____

_____   _____

_____   _____

_____   _____

_____   _____

_____   _____

_____   _____

The best office environments:

1. Keep distractions to a minimum.

2. Have good lighting with a minimum of glare.

3. Allow you to have control over your lighting, temperature, humidity.

4. Have a relative humidity of around 50 percent.

5. Allow you to see outside.

6. Have few distracting sounds.

7. Are ones where workers are considerate of each other.

Smoking Smoking remains a problem for many non-smoking workers. Many cities have now passed ordinances regulating smoking in office spaces. If smoke is distracting you on the job, you must do something about it. Putting up with conditions unacceptable to your good health and vitality is not only unproductive but can be dangerous. Studies have shown that ''passive'' smoking is harmful to your lungs.

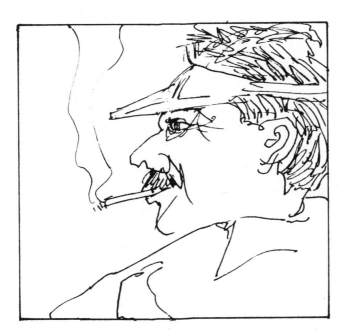

THE OFFICE ENVIRONMENT: A CHECK LIST

To identify potential problems in your office, take the time to complete the following check list:

Lighting types:

Building: _____

Office: _____

Full-spectrum lighting? No _____ Yes _____

Incandescent? No _____ Yes_____

Desk lamp with movable arm? No _____ Yes _____

Room:

Average temperature: _____

Average humidity: _____

Rate noise level: Quiet: _____ Some sound: _____ Noisy:_____

Very noisy: _____ Loud noise: _____ Background music: _____

Disturbing loud noises during the day: _____

Nearest distance from other workers: _____

Floor coverings: _____

Wall-covering materials: _____

Colors on walls: _____

Room size: _____

How many people in room: _____

Partitioned office spaces? No _____ Yes _____

Machines in vicinity:

Number within 10″: _____ 30″: _____ 100″: _____

Number of machines in your work station: _____

Is smoking allowed? No _____ Yes _____ If so, where? _____

YOUR WORKSTATION

Take Charge   You are the captain of this ship. Your office is your cabin to organize, maintain, run, live in, and operate. When you get into an automobile for the first time, you probably take a few minutes to adjust the seat, arrange the mirrors, and locate the turn signals before you drive off. Survey your workstation as a good captain would a ship. Here is where you earn your livelihood by performing vital tasks, ones important to your company. You also want to be kept safe and sound on your journey with your company. Make your workstation accommodate your physical and mental requirements so that you can do the best job possible.

Your company probably provided you with your workstation, but most companies do not tailor it to fit. It is up to you to make the needed alterations. You are either working at a new workstation or one that was previously occupied. When taking a new position with a company, you make certain changes at your desk automatically. The following guidelines will help provide yourself with the best environment possible under your particular circumstances.

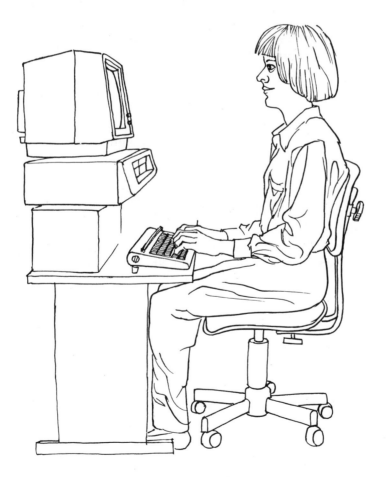

YOUR WORKSTATION (Continued)

Psychological Comfort   Take a careful look at your workstation. Pretend it's your first day on the job and you are moving into a space that someone else has vacated. Does it look inviting and comfortable, the sort of place you'll enjoy coming to each day? If not, change it. Add some pictures, a poster or two, even some flowers or a plant if company policy allows. Your psychological disposition affects your physical comfort. And when you feel good, you get more done.

Organize Your Work Surfaces   Check your work surfaces for messes that bother you. Clean up piles of papers that need to be filed, delegated, or discarded. Remember, your desk top is not a storage space. Your desk top should be reserved for papers and files that are being worked on. Everything else has a place; if it doesn't, create one. Have plenty of working surface on either side of your machine to lay out the papers or documents you're working on.

The Chair   Get your chair adjusted exactly the way you want it. Make sure that you always use the same well adjusted chair each day. Learn to identify "your" chair. Your chair should be adjusted to fit the contours and size requirements of your body in order to support good posture while you work. A lightly padded chair is best. Deep cushioned chairs are for lounging in your living room. Your body will tend to slide more on plastic covered chairs, and the plastic, which doesn't "breathe," can cause you to sweat. A nonslip, textured fabric or leather covering is ideal. It takes less effort to maintain good posture when you've got a good chair to sit on.

Use an adjustable, swivel moving chair on rollers with arm rests (unless you find arm rests get in your way). It is best if you can move your chair around freely. If your job requires a lot of movement across the floor in your chair, a chair with a five-legged base gives you more stability and is less likely to tilt back or tip over. Most new adjustable office chairs are the kind with a five-legged base on rollers. The base should extend beyond the perimeter of the seat. The heavier the user and the higher the chair seat, the larger this perimeter should be. High chair stools for facilitating meetings or for working at drafting tables, for example, should have a larger base perimeter than a desk chair.

Adjust the height of your chair seat so that your feet can rest flat on the floor or on your footstool. The front of the chair seat should be curved down and must not press on your upper legs, cutting off circulation. If the chair seat is too high, either adjust it down or get a foot rest. Adjust the seat pan forward if your work requires you to lean forward at your desk to read or write, but not so much that you slide forward. This will help you maintain the natural curve of your spine and reduce pressure on your thighs. If you operate a computer terminal and keyboard and your work does not require very much reading or writing, you will probably want your seat pan to be either flat or tilted slightly backward (not more than 5 degrees) to enable you to take more advantage of the lumbar support in the back rest.

Be sure that the backrest is adjusted to the natural curve of your spine when you are sitting with proper posture. Your chair should encourage you to sit with good posture. Slumped posture increases pressure on the discs between your vertebrae and makes your back muscles and ligaments work harder.

Arm rests are valuable supports for your forearms and help support the shoulders, upper body, and will even relieve stress on the neck. They also help you in getting up and sitting down.

Arm rests should usually be adjusted to between 7" and 11" above the seat. Some people prefer chairs without arm rests, but they can provide you with good upper body support.

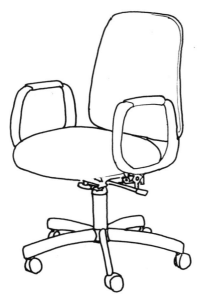

YOUR WORKSTATION (Continued)

The Work Surface   The key here is adjustability. Be sure that your work surface is adjusted for you. Check the height and depth of your table to make sure you have adequate leg room. Surface width must provide enough space for other desk top equipment such as a document holder, calculator, telephone, etc. A table with two different levels, one for the VDT and one for the keyboard, is often the most adaptable. Table height affects the height of the display and keyboard, which in turn affect your vision comfort, neck, back, and arms.

There are considerable differences in using typewriters and computers. Professional typists are more likely to look aside to regard text lying flat on a desk next to the typewriter or standing upright on a display stand. The VDT worker usually gazes straight ahead at a screen. Become aware of these postural differences and make the necessary adjustments. If you are using a typewriter, you may feel a little more comfortable with your forearms angled up just a bit. With the computer, the keyboard can be lower and the best forearm position is probably level with your elbows and the table. If you work at a desk writing or reading books, support your arms and elbows on the table as you work and you will probably want to lean forward.

Here are some general pointers regarding your working surface: Adjust your table height 3″ to 6″ above your lap for your keyboard. Use a higher level for the display terminal. Standard table heights are 28″ above the floor. Computer tables come with a keyboard shelf that is lower than 28″ from the floor. The depth of the table surface should be a minimum of 30″ to 36.″ A minimum 36″ table width is preferred. Check the surface for reflections. If necessary, lay down dark matte finish construction paper to cut glare.

Keyboard   Where you place your keyboard will depend on how extensively you use it. If it is central to your work, it will be located directly in front of you. If not, you may want to place it to one side. Being able to position your keyboard is essential. There are tactile and auditory keyboards, each providing feedback when a key is depressed. With the tactile key, generally preferred for high speed typing, you feel that the key has been pressed. The auditory keyboard provides a soft clicking sound. If the rear height is not adjustable on your keyboard, use a piece of wood to position it at exactly the right angle.

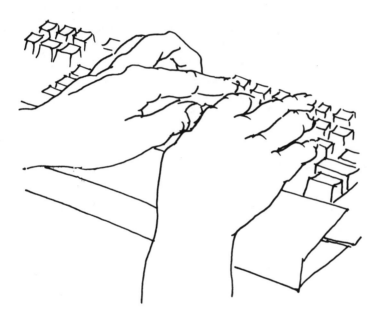

Hand Support   Writers, computer programmers, typesetters, data entry clerks, telephone operators, and administrative personnel who spend hours with their fingers in motion on a keyboard are prime candidates for repetitive motion injuries—the pain and swelling of carpal tunnel syndrome (CTS). Today's standard keyboards do not allow operators to rest their hands while typing. Over time the unsupported motion of the hands can cause swelling in the hands and arms, CTS, tenosynovitis, tendonitis, and bursitis. Early medical care is recommended if you are having these systoms.

A keyboard hand support can provide relief for people beginning to experience hand or finger pain, weakness, numbness and difficulty holding onto things. The support keeps the wrists and hands level and relaxed while they move. Sunflex makes a product called "Wrist Relief," a metal flange with a plastic foam pad on top that can be bent into the most comfortable position. It lies on the table in front of your keyboard.

YOUR WORKSTATION (Continued)

Footrest If your feet don't touch the floor comfortably, use a portable footrest that holds both feet and has a nonskid surface. The footrest should be heavy enough or stable enough not to move around under your feet.

Drafting Tables If you work at a drafting table, you will probably want the entire table top to be tilted toward you. Some tables using drafting machines are tilted almost vertical. Most, however, are only tilted 10 degrees or so. Be very careful if you sit on a high stool. Be sure that you have adequate foot support; don't rely on the rungs of the stool. A wooden or metal seat on a stool can be very uncomfortable after only a short time. Cushion your seat. I recommend using a stool that is fashioned like an adjustable chair so that you can adjust the seat height and backrest. Stand often, and while you work, support your arms on the drafting table. If you alternate between standing and sitting at a drafting table, be sure that you put one foot up on a footstool to elevate one leg at a time. This will help to keep the natural curvature of your lower lumber region and the pelvis tilted forward, a much less stressful position than if you stand with your weight equally distributed on the floor.

The general rule is the closer you have to use your eyes and hands together, the higher the work surface. That way, the arms, elbows, and upper body can be supported to the work surface without excessive leaning.

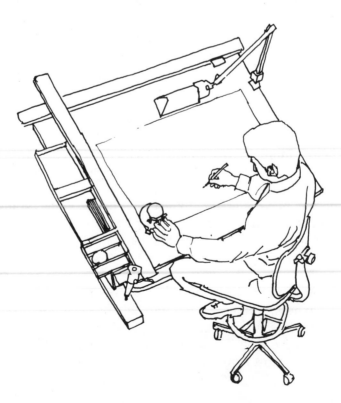

Location of Visual Display Terminals   The first criteria for VDT location is that characters and graphics be clearly visible, but keeping a distance of 24″ from the screen is recommended. You should be able to see the characters on your VDT without leaning your body forward or backward. The farther away you are from the screen, the less likely you will be affected by electromagnetic radiation. Although many articles have been written on VDT radiation danger, so far the evidence seems to be very controversial. See chapter on Long Term Concerns.

If the VDT is central to your work place, it is directly in front of you. Locate the top of the screen to be even with your eyes. If it must be higher than that, tilt it up at an angle so that the face of the screen is at a right angle and frontal to your line of sight.

If you are doing data entry, working from a hard copy, and only need the screen to check accuracy, position the hard copy on a stand in front of you with the keyboard on the table surface also directly in front of you. The screen can then be placed to one side and angled toward you.

If you read and write from your screen, place the screen facing you and your papers to one side or the other, depending which hand you write with. If you primarily read the screen and write from it and only occasionally use your keyboard, put the keyboard to the side and your writing materials on the table in front of the screen.

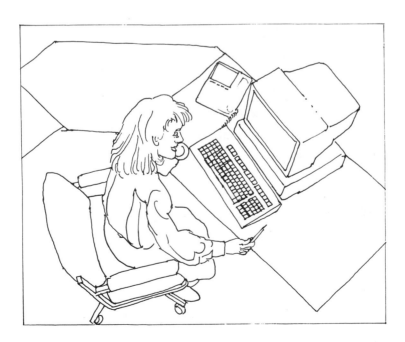

YOUR WORKSTATION (Continued)

Document Holder In general, place the document holder frontal to your vision as much a possible and to the right or left side of the display so that it, too, is perpendicular to your line of sight. Avoid awkward positions where you must work with your head turned in one direction or another. If you are doing data entry and you read from the document holder almost continuously, put it directly in front of you, just below the display screen; or move the display to one side and put the document straight ahead at the same level as the display. For data entry and retrieval, place the display and document side by side.

Other Tips Necessary reference books should be within reach without straining your body to reach them. If you are doing considerable referencing to one side of you, change to the other side every few hours or at least every few days. This will help to balance body movements and stretches.

Typewriter Tip If you work at a typewriter, alternate your reference work from side to side during the day. This will add natural stretching and balanced movement to your work positions. One woman had to have physical therapy for two years because she had always worked the entire day looking to her left. Beware of imbalanced activities. When we walk, we step on one foot then the other, always alternating. When we work, we must learn to do the same.

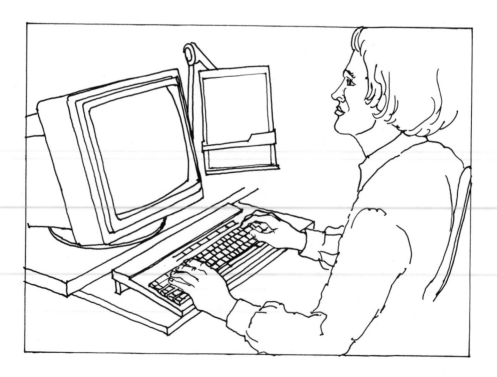

The Telephone   If you conduct business on the telephone each day, locate the telephone in an easy-to-reach place to the side of your workstation. In his book *Phone Power,* George Walther suggests that you keep a fresh notepad and a favored pen near your phone. He suggests that the phone place be a "sanctuary" kept apart from your other work. When an incoming call comes, you are always prepared and you won't have to disrupt your other work. If you don't have to write while speaking on the phone, use the interruption as an opportunity to stand up and stretch your legs. Speaking on the phone while standing will also put more life in your voice, giving the person on the line a stronger "voice picture" of you.

A Headset   A headset allows you to work with the telephone in greater comfort. It is ideal for people who conduct most of their business on the phone. Not just telephone company operators and switchboard operators, but also travel agents, receptionists, answering services, telemarketers, administrative assistants, and even executives will benefit. If you equip yourself with a headset, you can keep your hands free while on the phone to record key information, search files, write, and anything else you like. The habit of holding a telephone handset up to your ear with your shoulder so that you can use both hands to work can cause all kinds of neck and shoulder strain and upper back problems, guaranteeing a visit to your chiropractor. The habit of supporting the hand-held phone receiver with your elbow on the table can cause nerve pinching in the elbow as well as other complaints resulting from this unbalanced posture.

A headset allows you to sit or stand with a straight neck and spine while talking on the phone. It keeps your hands free to write, type, and search in file drawers. You can hear better with a headset. You can even gesture with your hands while talking, putting more emphasis in the voice picture you present over the phone. Headsets are so convenient that it is surprising more people don't use them.

YOUR WORKSTATION (Continued)

Clutter   Clutter can't hurt you too much physically, but, psychologically, it can be devastating to your peace of mind. Everything that is on your desk or work surface should be something you need to perform your job. When you are not using something, put it away where it belongs. Everything has a place. If it doesn't, it belongs in the waste basket. Unnecessary clutter adds chaos to your visual field and hides messages and important papers you really need. Pick up your clutter. Organize your work surface. Make an agreement to housekeep your workstation at the end of each day. Before you go home, put mess away or throw it away. Ask yourself, what do I use every day, once a week, once a month? Anything that you do not use every day gets put away, in a drawer, box, or shelf. Keep just the essentials in front of you. Position high use items close to you and the occasional use items within reach but further away. Once you have an organized desk, you will feel a lot better about your work space and about yourself.

Reducing Glare   To reduce eye strain and discomfort from glare on your screen, do the following:

1. Avoid bright lights shining directly on your monitor. Check your screen for reflections when it is turned off. Eliminate them as much as possible by adjusting the tilt (up and down) and the rotation (side to side) of the monitor.

2. If necessary, make a cardboard shield for the top and sides of the monitor. This shield will also allow you to reduce the brightness of the monitor image, which will also decrease the radiation.

3. Be sure that the monitor image is sharp, in perfect focus. Fuzzy images also cause eye strain.

4. Install a filter to reduce glare and reflections.

5. Keep your screen free of screen grime with regular dusting and cleaning.

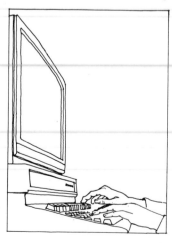

YOUR WORK STATION—CHECK LIST

Go through the following check list and become aware of your work environment. This is the first step to taking charge.

Lighting types:

In your office building: _____

In your work place: _____

At your desk: _____

Full-spectrum lighting? No _____ Yes _____

Incandescent? No _____ Yes _____

Desk lamp with a movable arm? No _____ Yes _____

Chair:

Are you comfortable in your chair? Yes _____ No _____

Seat height: _____ Fixed _____ Adjustable _____

Adjustable back: _____ On rollers _____ Swivel _____

Arm rests: _____ Do they fit your arms comfortably? _____

Chair seat covering material: _____

Table:

Table height: _____ Fixed _____ Adjustable _____

Size: _____ Large enough? _____

At desk:

Average temperature: _____

Average humidity: _____

Rate noise level: Quiet _____ Some sound _____ Noisy _____

Nearest distance from next desk: _____

Floor covering under chair and table: _____

Wall or partition covering material: _____

Colors on walls or partition: _____

Type of machine(s) you use: _____

Keyboard height: _____ Forearms horizontal? _____

Hands level? _____ Raised _____ Lower _____

YOUR WORKSTATION CHECKLIST (Continued)

Telephone location: _____   Headset: _____

Answering machine: _____   Message pad: _____

Calculator: _____   Rolodex: _____   Container for pens and pencils: _____

Disk files: _____   In/Out trays: _____   Clock visible: _____

List other equipment: _____

_____

Distance you can see from your work station: _____

Interior window: Size: _____

Nearest exterior window: Size: _____   Distance from desk: _____

Describe the indoor view from your desk: _____

_____

_____

Describe the outdoor view: _____

_____

_____

Machines in vicinity:

VDT's   Number within 10″ _____   30″ _____   100″ _____

Other   Number within 10″ _____   30″ _____   100″ _____

Number of machines in your work station: _____

How private is your workstation?

Very private: _____   Somewhat private: _____   Not at all private: _____

Sound privacy?

Very private: _____   Somewhat private: _____   Not at all private: _____

Visual privacy?

Very private: _____   Somewhat private: _____   Not at all private: _____

_____

Visual Display Terminal No. 1:

Distance between screen and eyes: _____

Screen colors: Background: _____ Symbols: _____

Reflections on screen? No: _____ Yes: _____ Sources: _____

_____

Screen filter? No: _____ Yes: _____ Type: _____

Visual Display Terminal No. 2:

Distance between screen and eyes: _____

Screen colors: Background: _____ Symbols: _____

Reflections on screen? No: _____ Yes: _____ Sources: _____

_____

Screen filter? No: _____ Yes: _____ Type: _____

Visual Display Terminal No. 3:

Distance between screen and eyes: _____

Screen colors: Background: _____ Symbols: _____

Reflections on screen? No: _____ Yes: _____ Sources: _____

_____

Screen filter? No: _____ Yes: _____ Type: _____

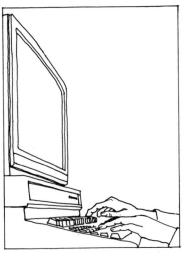

MY WORKSTATION SET-UP

A Promissory Contract

By: _____ (Date)

I _____ will check my workstation set-up.

I promise to: (Check those you currently do or plan to initiate within the next week).

☐ 1. Make my workstation an inviting place to work, for my psychological and physical comfort.

☐ 2. Reduce clutter and clean up papers that need to be filed, delegated, or discarded each day.

☐ 3. Remember that my desk top is a work space, not a storage space.

☐ 4. Use a comfortable, well adjusted movable chair or stool on rollers.

☐ 5. Check my chair seat height adjustment each day so that my feet can rest comfortably on the floor.

☐ 6. Place a footrest under my work surface if I sit on a stool or my feet don't reach the floor comfortably.

☐ 7. Adjust my table top height.

☐ 8. Consider tilting my work surface forward to allow for more comfort.

☐ 9. Make the top of my screen even with my eyes.

☐ 10. Organize the equipment on top of my desk according to its frequency of use.

☐ 11. Keep frequently used reference materials within reach.

☐ 12. Alternate my reference work from side to side.

☐ 13. Create a special place for the telephone with appropriate notetaking materials.

☐ 14. Use a headset if I am on the phone more than off.

☐ 15. Guard against interruptions and eliminate possible opportunities for eye contact from my workstation with people in public corridors.

☐ 16. Sit on the seat of my chair with my weight forward and off my spine. I may need to get a small wedge cushion on my chair seat to do this.

☐ 17. Sit so that my eyes are no closer than 24″ from the surface of my screen.

☐ 18. Be sure that my chair allows free movement so that I can keep moving and taking my mini-breaks through the day.

☐ 19. Check my screen for reflections and do what is necessary to eliminate all the reflections from my screen.

☐ 20. Get a glare filter for my screen to insure the best possible contrast and keep reflections from distracting my vision.

☐ 21. Keep the machine and desk top dusted and clean. If it is appropriate, I will keep a feather duster in my drawer.

☐ 22. Be sure that I can look at least 20″ into the distance to rest my eyes.

☐ 23. Put up a landscape poster on the wall—a beach, forest, or some pleasing natural environment—an image that is relaxing and inviting will be the most beneficial.

Signed _____
                     (your signature)

YOUR BODY

Now that you have become aware of your physical environment, it is time to become aware of your physical body. Realize that those little or big pains you have been putting up with over the years just don't have to be there. But where *are* they? Over the next few days, make a thorough examination of your body. How do you feel at different times of the day? Where do you hurt? Where are you stiff? Are your joints sore? Do you have muscle stiffness? Are you experiencing nerve pain? Are you experiencing numbness? Use the following check list to make your investigation.

Describe your symptoms and their location.

Body Discomfort—describe frequency and intensity:

Head
Headache _____
Eye strain _____
Burning eyes _____
Dry eyes _____
Blurry vision _____
Dry mouth _____

Neck
Stiff neck _____
Neck pain _____
Limited movement _____
Tightness in the neck _____

Shoulders
Shoulder pain _____
Shoulder stiffness _____

Back
Upper back pain _____
Tightness in the upper back _____
Stiffness in the upper back _____
Lower back pain _____
Tightness in the lower back _____
Stiffness in the lower back _____
Lower backache _____

Abdomen

Stomach pain _____

Heartburn _____

Intestinal gas _____

Stomach disorders _____

Digestive problems _____

Constipation _____

Legs

Upper leg aches and/or pains _____

Lower leg aches and/or pains _____

Numbness _____

Nerve pain _____

Stiffness in the legs _____

Leg cramps _____

Feet

Foot pain _____

Foot cramps _____

Arms

Sore elbows _____

Numbness _____

Hands

Numbness _____

Pain in the hands or fingers _____

If any of the above symptoms persist, see your health practitioner immediately.

YOUR HABITS

Most physical discomfort can be avoided by eliminating the *habits* that cause physical and mental stress and establishing habits that further mental and physical health and well-being. The following section will help you establish your motivations for change, increase your awareness of the habits that do not further your well-being, and assist you in establishing the habits and procedures that can make your work more productive and comfortable.

First, we must become aware of what we are doing that keeps us from our optimum productivity. Based upon your reading so far, list the habits that inhibit your optimum performance.

HABIT LIST

1.

2.

3.

4.

5.

6.

HABITS: HOW TO CHANGE THEM

When we work, we very quickly establish habits. Some are helpful and some are not. When we identify which habits are beneficial and which aren't, we can then proceed to eliminate the ones we don't want and replace them with better ones. It is not enough just to stop doing something. For example, if you are a smoker and want to change that habit, you transform yourself from being an habitual smoker—one who breathes in smoke during certain times every day—to a person who breathes in air at all times. You change from thinking of yourself as a smoke breather to thinking of yourself as an air breather. To do this, you must change how you think of yourself. The easiest way to change a habit is to replace it with another habit. So we will replace undesirable habits with desirable ones.

There are six steps involved in changing a habit.

1. Identify the habit

2. Know the alternative(s)

3. Desire one alternative

4. Choose the alternative

5. Change thinking or beliefs to allow the new mental set

6. Practice the alternative thinking and action until it is an established habit; this usually takes three to four weeks.

Don't skip ahead to step six without first completing steps 1–5. First we become aware of undesirable habits. Then we decide how we will replace them.

Using the previous list, prioritize the primary undesirable habits that you would like to change. Then list their desirable replacement.

UNDESIRABLE HABITS　　　　　**DESIRABLE HABITS**

1. _____　_____

2. _____　_____

3. _____　_____

4. _____　_____

5. _____　_____

6. _____　_____

FITNESS AT THE DESK: *SITTING*

Who ever would have thought that sitting could be hazardous to our health? And yet typical hazards from sitting all day include weak abdominal muscles, weak thighs, constipation, sore or stiff neck, stiff back, lower back pain, poor circulation, and overweight, to name the most common. It may sound strange, but our bodies were not designed to be sitting in chairs. It is much more natural to stand, squat, lie, or sit cross-legged on the ground. But the chair appears to be here to stay. So sit we must. See Your Work Station, for advice on how to make your chair provide proper support.

When we sit, our abdominal muscles relax and our front and inner thighs and buttock muscles become inactive. Therefore, it is important that these muscles get special attention on the job and during your exercise program. Here are some recommended exercises you can do while sitting at your desk.

BLTs Tighten your buttock muscles. You will feel yourself rise in your chair a bit, hold, and then lower yourself again by relaxing the buttock muscles gently. Breathe in as you tighten, hold, and exhale as you let go.

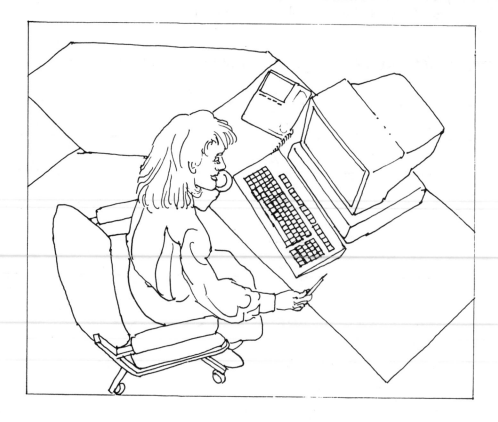

The Inner Thigh Press

Straighten your arms with your fists together. Place your fists between your knees. Now press your legs together hard agaist your fists. Hold for the count of 4 and relax. Inhale as you push, hold, and exhale as you relax.

Knee Lifts

Push back from desk so that you knees clear the edge of the table. Raise knee as high as you can. Hold for the count of 4 and then slowly lower it. Alternate legs. Breathe in through your nose as you raise your knee, hold breath for the count of four, and exhale through your mouth as you lower your knee. A variation: Lift the knee as high as you can; then pull it toward your chest with your hands for a final stretch.

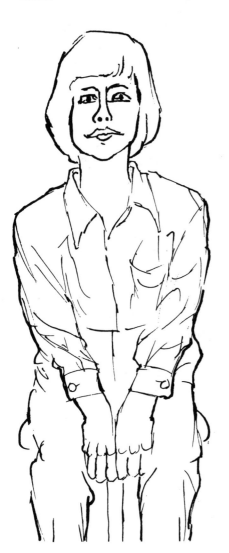

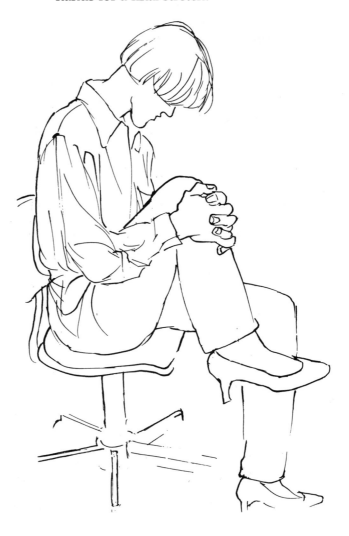

FITNESS AT THE DESK: *SITTING*

MOVEMENT PROMOTES ALIVENESS—Ways To Add Movement On The Job

"Life is movement, movement is life."

If there is one idea that will improve the way you feel, it is "move more!" The author of a book on Hatha Yoga claims that health and longevity depend on the flexibility of the spine. This may be true, but health also requires the flexibility of all parts of the body. It is through movement that we stay flexible. It is with movement that the body stays healthy. The heart beats, the blood flows, the lungs move in and out, the muscles expand and contract. The more movement that we can integrate into our workday, the better we will feel. Sitting at a desk can be detrimental to your body if you don't keep moving. Here are some ways to add movement to your body while sitting. Most of these can be done as a normal part of your work.

Movement while sitting

Wings Put your arms straight out as if they were wings. Do not lock your elbows. Keep your hands and fingers open and relaxed. Rotate your arms in tight circles forwards, then backwards with your palms facing the floor. Put your arms down. Breathe in and out once, then repeat, this time with your palms facing forwards. Put your arms down. Breathe in and out again; then repeat with the palms facing the ceiling. Put your arms down. Breathe in and out again, and then repeat with the palms facing in back of you. Put your arms down and breathe.

Shoulder Rolls Roll your shoulders back, up, forward, and down—five times. Then reverse, roll your shoulders forward, up, back and down—five times. Finally, lift the shoulders up as if trying to touch the ears. Then relax them and let them fall. Inhale and exhale with each of these moves. These moves can be done while you are reviewing data on the screen.

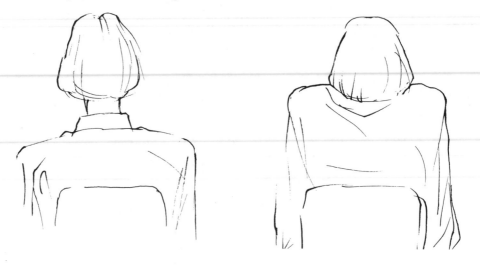

Head Movement   Neck and shoulder tightness can be alleviated if you will learn to move your head as you read. Children do this naturally when they learn to read. Some of us were taught that this is wrong. We were told to keep our heads still and we were trained to let only the eyes move back and forth. Whether you are reading a typed hard copy or a visual display terminal, move your head back and forth as it naturally feels comfortable. You will notice an immediate relaxation of the eyes, neck, and shoulders when you do.

Head Flops   While you wait for your machine to complete a command, let your head flop gently from side to side, then down toward your chest and back. I don't believe in neck rolls. I think this can cause problems. Just the side to side and forward to back motion is enough. Doing this often will keep the neck flexible and the eyes relaxed. It will also help with occasional and chronic headaches.

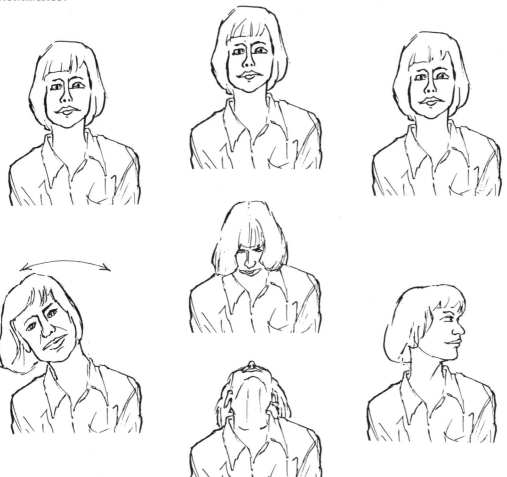

FITNESS AT THE DESK: *SITTING*

The Roll Down   Push yourself away from your desk with arms relaxed and hanging to your sides. Begin by rolling your head down, touch your chin to your chest, and continue to roll down until your head is well between your legs and your hands and arms are hanging down toward the floor. Then, slowly roll back up again, using your leg muscles. Do not push yourself up with your arms. Exhale as you roll down and inhale as you roll back up. You will feel the stretch in the neck, upper back, and lower back. This roll also increases circulation in the head, eyes, and brain.

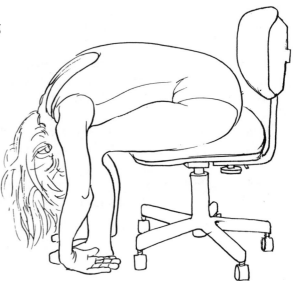

Back Front Push   Sitting with your back straight, bring your hands up level with your shoulders. Using your upper arms, push back as if you are trying to get your shoulder blades to touch each other. Then bring your hands together in front of you still at shoulder height. Put your palms together and push, hold for a slow count of five, and relax.

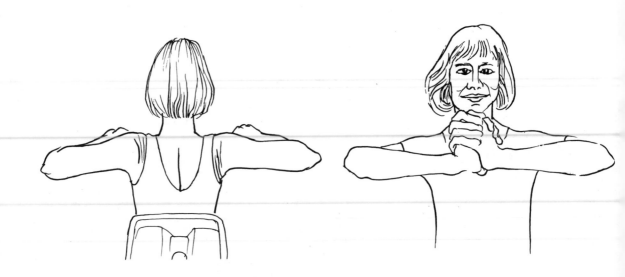

FITNESS AT THE DESK: *STANDING*

The Long Swing   This is a very relaxing traditional vision care movement. Stand with your feet about 18" apart, and slowly swing your upper body around and look behind you first in one direction, then in another. Allow your arms and hands to swing with complete relaxation as your body moves back and forth. Lift the heel of the opposite foot off the floor as you swing. Breathe deeply as you swing and blink regularly as you passively view the room moving in the opposite direction. Enjoy the relaxed movement. Do this as long as you like. Fifty times before bed at night will keep your eyes relaxed while you sleep.

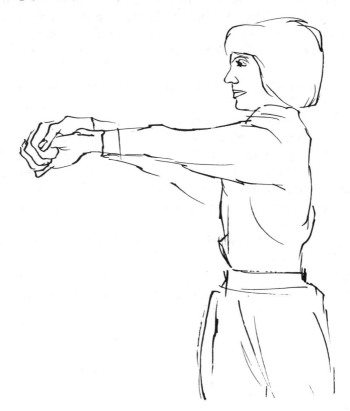

The Standing Upper Body Swing   Raise arms as if you are going to rest them on a shelf in front of you at shoulder level. Rest the palm of one hand on the back of the other. Now swing to the right as far as you can go. Now move yourself a little further—stretching your sides and back—and repeat 10 times. Return to the front and now swing to the left and again stretch 10 times. Your head must follow your body in this one. Look off to the distance with relaxed vision as you perform these motions.

The movements described above can be done intermittently throughout the day.

R AND R—REST AND RELAXATION DURING THE DAY

One important attitude to gain and maintain is the attitude of relaxation. It involves the simple habit of mentally suggesting to yourself, "Relax." When you do this, you will feel a "letting go" in the body and a "letting go" with your mind. You become much more willing to understand opposing points of view. You have a greater capacity to accept your environment and the people around you without negative, destructive thoughts. When you feel your body relax, you will also feel a letting go with your mind. A relaxed mind and body can contribute to a long and happy life. Relaxation on the job is very important. Work situations can be very stressful. Learning the habit of relaxation can transform your experience of your work environment.

Here are a number of suggestions for keeping relaxed during the day.

Leave Enough Time   Leave home early enough to arrive at work early. If you have the habit of arriving late to work, realize that this is getting the day off to a stressed beginning. Even if no one knows the difference, you do. Break that pattern now and give yourself a break. You most likely feel guilty about being late. Leave in plenty of time so that you won't have to race to work. Plan your departure so that you will arrive 15 minutes early, without hurrying.

In order to arrive at work 15 minutes early, I must leave by _____ .

Let Go   Get into the habit of letting go. When you feel your breathing restricted and your stomach turn inside out, consciously suggest to your body to let go.

Take Sitting-down Breaks   Every 15 minutes, stop, stretch, and do some of the sitting-down movements described on pages 48–52.

Take Stand-up Breaks   Every 15 minutes, stop, stand up, stretch, and sit down again. This will help you keep your muscles relaxed.

Take Non-Coffee Breaks   At coffee break, instead of drinking coffee, have herb tea or close your eyes for a few minutes. Do some breathing exercises. Go for a brisk walk outside your building. It will be a lot more refreshing than a cup of coffee.

Lunch Time—Relax Time   Make lunch a time to relax. Eat a light lunch and stay away from coffee and alcohol. Some people use their lunch hour to exercise. The Italians take a long lunch period and go home and sleep. It's not a bad idea but hardly practical in the United States. Lying down can be very rejuvenating if you can manage it in your corporate environment without criticism.

Eyes-Closed Breathing   The afternoon break is even more important than the morning break. This is the time to relax with the eyes closed and do 10 deep breathing exercises.

Working Overtime   If on certain days you must work late, be sure to have a light supper, again with no coffee or alcohol. Meditate or lie down before you continue into the night.

Sleep   Get a good night's sleep. To be productive, we need to be fully rested.

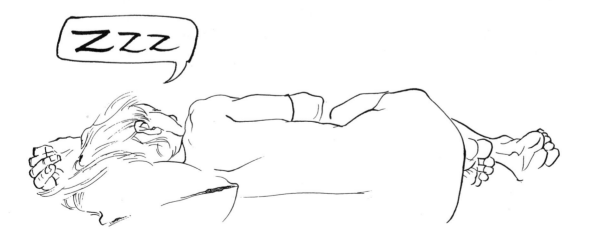

BREATHING FOR LIFE

Oxygen affects the quality of life of every cell in your body. Fully oxygenating your system at various times during the day will keep your cells happy and your body feeling good. Deep diaphragmic breathing is the way to do this. This is how it is done.

1. Begin by exhaling through your mouth all your air so that you can begin with all fresh air.

2. Relax your stomach and lower diaphragm muscles. Let the air naturally inflate your diaphragm from the bottom up, breathing in through your nose.

3. Keep on inflating. You will feel your chest and rib cage expand as you fill your lungs. As your lungs fill, be careful not to draw your diaphragm inward.

4. After you have inhaled completely, exhale gently and slowly through your mouth. Don't let the air come rushing out. Instead, control the air as it flows out. Relax your chest and rib cage while you exhale.

5. Finally, pull your diaphragm in to empty the last bit of air through your mouth. Be careful not to slouch forward as you do this. Now you are ready to inhale again.

Deep breathing is best if you do it in this ratio: Inhale for a count of two, hold for eight counts, and exhale four counts. By exhaling more slowly, you eliminate the toxins in your body by way of the lymphatic system. When you hold for the count of eight you fully oxygenate the blood and activate your lymphatic system.

Deep breathing can done sitting at your desk or lying down. In either case, the process will be enhanced if you close your eyes and become aware of what your body is doing as you breathe. Relax your face, eyes, hands, and feet. Feel the subtle energy of this life-giving substance entering and leaving your body. Ideally, you should practice for five minutes three times a day. If you do deep breathing in the late afternoon when you begin to feel tired, you will notice you will feel refreshed and energized afterward.

The effectiveness of all the body movement exercises in this book will be greatly enhanced if you accompany them with deep breathing.

WRISTS, HANDS, AND FINGERS

It is important that we keep our wrists, hands, and fingers limber, relaxed, and strong. Finger pains, tingling hands, numbness, carpal tunnel syndrome (a condition in which tendons in the wrist become inflamed and pinch nerves), and repetitive motion syndrome can reduce your productivity and even incapacitate you as a VDT worker. Take a moment and look at your hands. Appreciate the job they do. What marvelous tasks they can perform! All hands are different; yet most keyboards are similar. As much as possible, adapt your keyboard to fit your hands by tilting it toward you or moving it forward or backward. Most hand and wrist problems are caused by the sequences of motion, repeated thousands of times, poor circulation, upper body pressure, and restrictive movement. If you are a telephone operator, travel agent, secretary, typist, computer operator, or do a lot of key fingering each day, be careful to treat your wrists, hands, and fingers with the love and attention they deserve. Most problems can be avoided with care for hands, wrists, and fingers, which includes proper position, movement, and stretches.

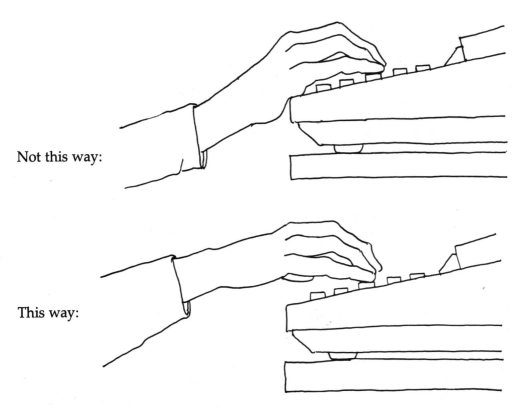

Not this way:

This way:

When using a keyboard or typewriter be careful not to let your hands rest on angled protrusions.

WRISTS, HANDS AND FINGERS (Continued)

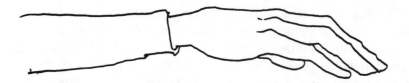

Position   The hands and wrists should be held in "the neutral positon"—a straight forward position. The wrist is not bent upwards or downwards or tilted one way or the other. Abnormal or bent wrist positions will be felt in the muscles, tendons, blood vessels, and nerves of the forearms, the upper arms, the shoulders, and even in the neck. The new machines are so sensitive that it takes almost no pressure to type. That means that you can keep your hands relaxed even while you work. The keyboard itself should be positioned so that your hand can work in the neutral position with the upper arms vertical and the forearms horizontal. People with long fingers tend to need the keys in a flat position, and people with short fingers may want the keyboard to be more inclined toward them. Some people type with their fingers almost straight, whereas others type with the fingers curved and rounded.

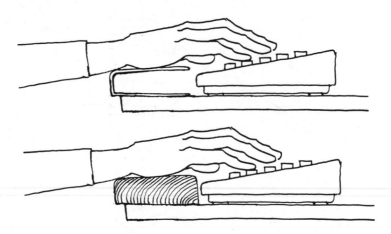

Wrist Rest   If you are using some kind of rest for your hand or wrist, be sure that it is soft, comfortable, and adjusted to your body. Don't ever put constant pressure or upper body weight on your wrists or forearms.

Repetitive Hand Movement   If your work requires mostly repetitive movement with the hands, it will be essential that you compensate for this by resting and doing alternate movements when your hands are off the keyboard. Here are some suggestions.

The Hand Shake   Simply dangle your fingers to your sides and shake your hand as you consciously relax your fingers. Your fingers will flop around loosely. This relaxes tight muscles and puts a fresh supply of blood into your fingers, hands, and wrists. Do this while you review material on your screen, as you walk, while on your break, and any time you think of it. Just 10 seconds of this movement will be very beneficial.

Spaghetti Fingers   This is a more active variation on the hand shake. It is best to do this standing away from furniture. Let your fingers dangle relaxed and then gently shake them back and forth, allowing them to flop around freely. Slowly raise your arms up until they are over your head, reaching for the ceiling. Continue to shake the hands on the way up and then on the way down. Time: about one minute.

Here are some of the stretching and moving exercises you can do to keep hands loose, relaxed, and flexible.

Finger Spread   Make your hands into a tight fist. Relax the fist and spread your fingers out, pushing them as far as they will go. Repeat five times. This stretch is best when your arms are hanging down toward the floor. Then gravity assists the blood flow into your fingers.

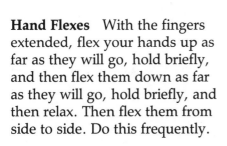

Hand Flexes   With the fingers extended, flex your hands up as far as they will go, hold briefly, and then flex them down as far as they will go, hold briefly, and then relax. Then flex them from side to side. Do this frequently.

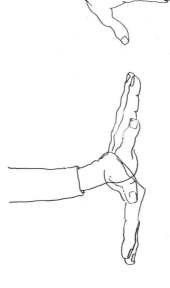

WRISTS, HANDS, AND FINGERS (Continued)

Wrist Stretch   This is a more aggressive stretch and must be used carefully. Put your right elbow on the table with your forearm vertical. With the left hand, *gently* pull the hand back toward the forearm by applying mild pressure on the palm and then gently push the hand forward by applying mild pressure on the back of your hand. Do the same thing with the left hand. Be very sensitive to any slight pain with this stretch. It must be done with care.

Because these movements and stretches are new, they may cause some discomfort at first. If after a few weeks these symptoms persist, consult a specialist.

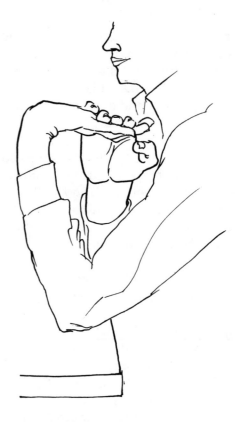

Awareness is the Key   As with all of the information in this book, daily awareness is the key to overcoming difficulties. Become aware of how your hands and arms are feeling with everything you do. Pay attention to any numbness or discomfort. Some exercises on your off hours that require hand and wrist work can also cause problems. Playing tennis, lifting and pulling weight, doing aerobics that require holding dumbells, running with weight in your hands, bicycle riding, push-ups, and baseball are all examples. Be aware of these and organize your exercise program to compensate for your work stresses.

LEG AND FOOT CARE

Chair Height The feet are farthest from the heart and need extra help in keeping good circulation. Common foot complaints include numbness, cramps, cold feet, and sore or tight muscles. The most common cause of these symptoms is the height of the chair seat. If your chair seat is too high and your feet cannot rest flat on the floor, then the blood flow to your feet is restricted by the pressure of the chair seat under your thighs. Habitual leaning in one direction can also place pressure on one thigh. Arrange your work surface so your posture is balanced.

Abnormal Leg Positions Problems can occur when your legs and feet are crossed. This not only cuts off circulation to the leg crossed but also twists the spine into an abnormal position. Abnormal leg positions will make you ache and can result in pinched nerves and cramped muscles.

Movement The more you move your legs and feet, the better. While sitting, move your feet up and down with your legs outstretched. Bring your weight forward and back as you sit. Move your feet in and out. Don't store items under your work space; leave room for your feet.

Standing Stand frequently. Walk around as much as possible. Some people prefer to work while standing. If you have adjusted your work surface for standing be sure that you have a foot stool under your table to rest and elevate one leg. Standing on both feet for long periods will stress the lower back.

Pockets Make sure that your back pockets are empty. Wallets or notebooks stuffed in your back pocket will change the level of your hips and restrict circulation.

Calves and Ankles Stand with your feet 12" apart and hold the back of your chair. Raise up on your toes as high as you can, keeping your body in perfect standing posture. Hold for the count of four, and then slowly lower your heels to the floor. Inhale as you raise and exhale as you lower yourself.

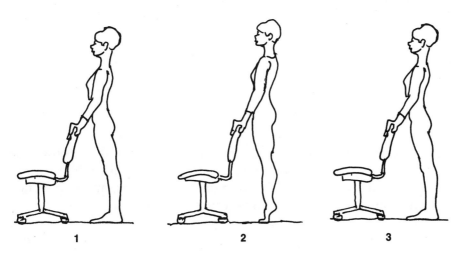

1   2   3

STRETCHING

Stretching keeps your body limber as you grow older. If you stretch every day, you can maintain your flexibility all your life. In my hometown of Madison, Wisconsin, there was a man who stretched, walked, and performed yoga exercises every day; he lived to be 99 years old. Yoga postures are the basis for many stretching exercises in the West. A routine of yoga in the morning and evening will do wonders for your health, circulation, and flexibility. If you don't think you have the time for yoga, there are stretching maneuvers you can do at the workstation that will keep you limber. When you do them, begin by telling yourself to "let go." Always breathe diaphragmically, as you stretch your muscles need oxygenated blood.

Side to Side Interlock your hands and thumbs together. Raise them high above your head—as high as you can. Facing forward, slowly swing your outstretched arms over to the right, stretching your left side. Then swing to the left, stretching the right side. Repeat one more time, then bring your arms down and shake your hands to relax them.

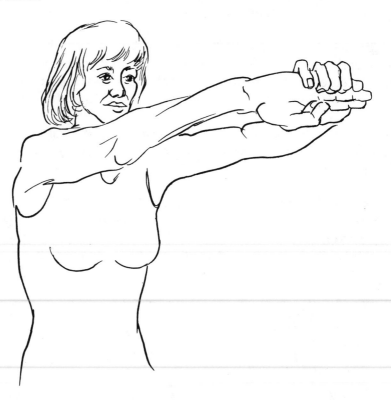

Arm and Upper Body Stretch Hold the back of one hand with the other and push your arms straight out in front of you as far as they will go. Now move your hand from side to side stretching your arms, shoulders, and upper chest. You can do this often, sitting or standing, during the day.

Upper Arm Stretch Put right arm up over your head and bring your hand down and place between your shoulder blades. Grasp your right elbow with your left hand and pull it further back, stretching your upper arm muscles. Repeat with the left arm.

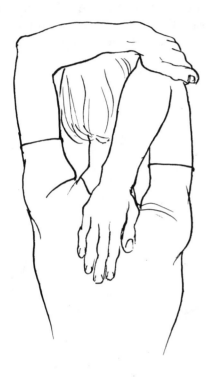

Body Twist Sitting with both feet on the floor, place both hands on the outside of your right thigh. Turn your head and upper torso to the right and look behind you, hold for five or six seconds and then face your desk. Don't strain but *do* stretch. Then twist to the left by placing your hands on the outside of the left thigh and turning your upper body around to look behind you, again holding for five or six seconds and then returning to the front. Inhale as you twist and exhale as you return to the front.

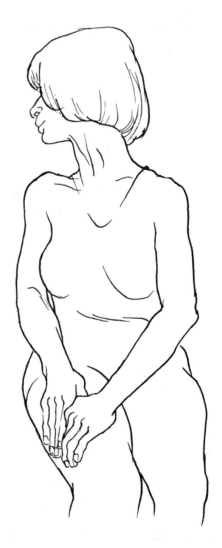

STRETCHING (Continued)

The Standing Roll Down   Stand with your arms hanging relaxed at your sides. Begin rolling your head down, touch your chin to your chest, and continue to roll down slowly until your head is as low as it will go. Let your arms and hands hang loosely toward the floor. Feel the force of gravity pulling you down. Do not lock your knees. Then, slowly roll back up again the same way you rolled down. This is an excellent maneuver to stretch and loosen the back and neck, and it will also increase circulation in the head, eyes, and brain. A very refreshing movement.

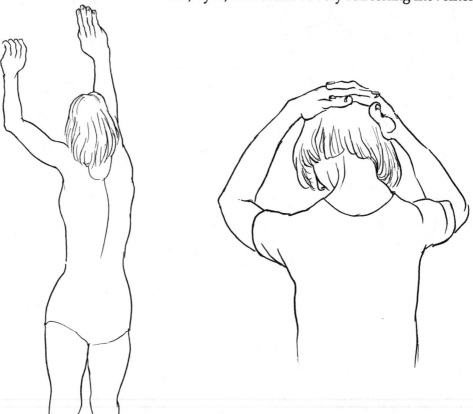

Reach For The Sky   Standing raise your arms above your head, alternating first one then the other to see how high you can reach. Shift your weight from one side to the other as you move upward. Visually look at the back of your hands and then up at the ceiling as fast as possible. Inhale through your nose as you stretch, then exhale through the mouth. If you can manage a yawn with this stretch, all the better.

Neck Stretch   Clasp hands on the back of your head. Drop your head forward so that your chin is close to the front of your neck. Relax your arms. That is enough. Don't try and pull your head down with your arms. Let the weight of your head and arm stretch your neck. Now rotate your head from side to side in this position. Do this stretch gently. At first you may want to use part of your arm weight to pull your head down.

EXERCISE

The body is a dynamically flexible, moving organism. Exercise keeps it that way. In some professions, from football to outside gardening, exercise is just part of the job. But for desk workers, exercise must be scheduled into the day. Regular exercise, along with proper nutrition, will preserve your energy for life. Sleep will help, but exercise will insure a high energy level. Proper exercise helps us to keep our muscle tone, maintain our correct body weight, rid our bodies of toxins and poisons, cleanse the pores of our skin with perspiration, keep our bones strong, exercise our heart muscle, cleanse the digestive and circulation system. This list could be continued, for exercise confers almost countless health benefits. In fact, there are so many benefits to regular exercise that it is alarming that so many people don't exercise regularly!

Walking from the apartment or house to the car, from the car to the office, and back again, is all the exercise some people get. Everyone knows people who have energy to spare. Ask them what they do for exercise, and you will probably find that they walk, jog, run, swim, trampoline, perform aerobics, or work out at a corporate fitness center or gym on a daily basis. They look great and usually have a sunny disposition. Personal and corporate productivity will increase if a regular program of physical exercise is followed. Exercise is just as important as sleep, food, and recreation. If you are not now following a regular daily exercise program, commit to one today.

Start out slowly if it has been a long time since you worked out. Be sure to get the approval of your doctor before you embark on a new exercise program.

Exercise each day for a minimum of one-half hour. You will most likely find that your productivity on the job increases. The time it takes to exercise will be time saved rather than time wasted. You will live longer and feel better each day. You will never, ever regret it.

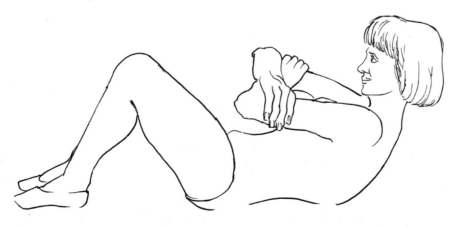

CONTRACT

Here is what I intend to do and when I intend to do it each day of the week.

DAY	TIME	TYPE OF EXERCISE
Monday	_____	_____
		_____
		_____
Tuesday	_____	_____
		_____
		_____
Wednesday	_____	_____
		_____
		_____
Thursday	_____	_____
		_____
		_____
Friday	_____	_____
		_____
		_____
Saturday	_____	_____
		_____
		_____
Sunday	_____	_____
		_____
		_____

MOVEMENT EXERCISES FOR PEOPLE WHO SIT AT WORK

There are many very well thought out exercise programs described in books and demonstrated on video cassette. Most exercise programs are aimed at weight loss or redistribution, muscle toning, and making your body beautifully proportioned. The main focus in this chapter is to teach you the movements you need to *feel* good, to eliminate the aches and pains that you may now experience.

If you are overweight, it is important for you to return to your recommended weight by a combination of diet and exercise. An overweight body takes more energy to maintain. This means you have less energy and vitality to put into your daily activities. Excess weight can also cause many physical ailments, leaving you less efficient and productive.

Following are a few movements that are particularly beneficial to people who sit at work. These movements will tone the parts of the body that do not get a workout. At first, do each as many times as you feel will benefit you. As you get stronger, increase the number of repetitions; the repetitions suggested are only a starting number. If you work-out continuously, you should be able to finish all of this program in 10 minutes.

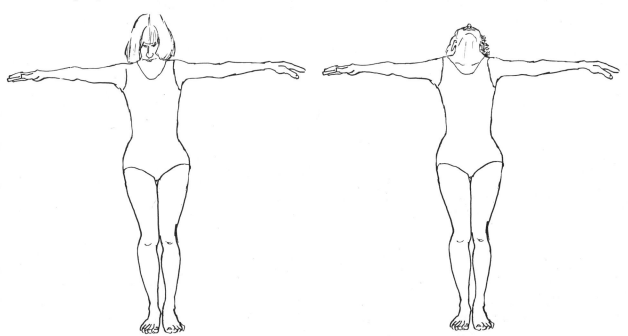

Head Drop Standing or sitting straight and tall with your arm and hands extended out to the sides at shoulder height, drop your head forward and down as far as it will go, then bring it back as far as it will go. *8 times*

MOVEMENT EXERCISES FOR PEOPLE
WHO SIT AT WORK (Continued)

Head Tilt   Sitting or standing with the arms hanging relaxed at your sides and looking forward, tilt your head from side to side as far as it will go.

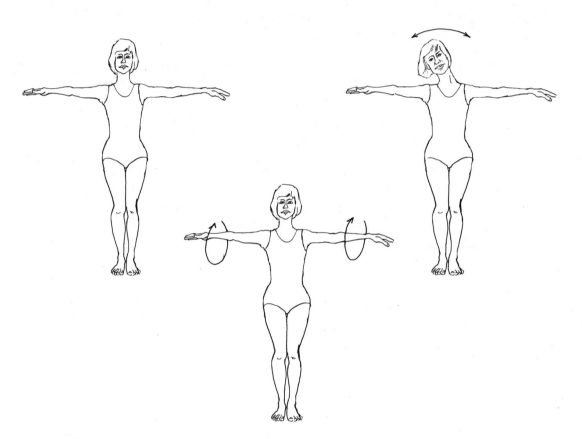

Arm Swings   Standing straight and tall, swing your arms forward, up, and around. *Keep your arms, hands and fingers relaxed.*   Then reverse the direction.
8 times each direction

Elbow Arm Stretch   Stand tall with your feet 12″ apart, your bent elbows held at shoulder height. Swing your elbows back as far as they will go, return, then swing whole arms back as far as they will go and return. Be careful not to lock elbows as the arms go back—keep the arms slightly bent. Make your hands into loose fists and maintain your arms at shoulder height as you move.
8 times

Arms to the Back   Sitting or standing tall with your arms straight at your sides and relaxed, move your arms back as far as they will go. Now push them further
10 times.

Doorway Push   Standing tall in an open doorway, place the backs of your hands against the jamb. Breathe in, hold, and push against the jamb hard, release, and exhale. *5 times*

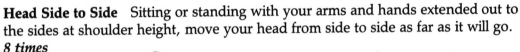

Side Stretch   Standing straight and tall, place your right hand up over your head and relax. Put your left hand on your hip. Lean to the left side as far as you can, and then move in very small movements, stretching even further. Then reverse. *20 times each side*

Head Side to Side   Sitting or standing with your arms and hands extended out to the sides at shoulder height, move your head from side to side as far as it will go. *8 times*

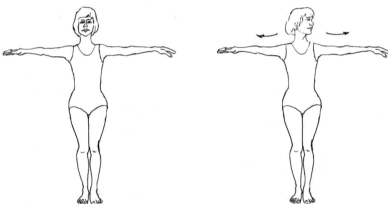

Leg Lifts   On all fours, bring the right knee up as close to your right ear as possible. Put your head down to try to meet your right knee. Then, slowly push your foot back and up as far as you can, arching your back and bringing your head back at the same time. *Repeat 8 times. Then repeat with the left leg 8 times.*

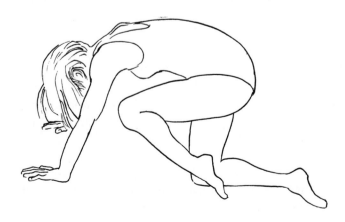

MOVEMENT EXERCISES FOR PEOPLE
WHO SIT AT WORK (Continued)

Tummy Tucker Lying on your back with the legs bent and the knees up, hold your elbows, take a deep breath, and exhale as you raise your head and shoulders off the floor and try to touch your forearms to your knees. Maintaining this position, work forward 10 times as if you are trying to advance your arms closer to the knees. Then relax and breathe in, lowering your head and shoulders to the floor. *Repeat 8 times.* Proper breathing is an important part of this exercise.

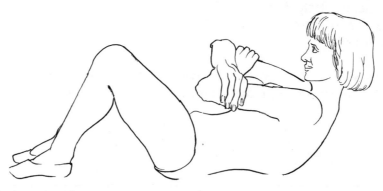

Plow Variation Lie flat on your back, arms at your sides, palms facing down on the mat. Breathe deeply once and relax. Without bending your legs, slowly raise your feet, legs, and hips off the floor as you inhale. When your legs are perpendicular with the floor, exhale and relax, with your feet pulled toward your head as far as possible. Inhale again, and then, as you exhale, slowly lower your feet to the floor in back of your head. Remain in this position for a few seconds, breathing normally through the nose, moving your feet back as far as you can and giving your neck a good stretch. While inhaling, return your legs to a perpendicular position. Then, as your exhale, slowly lower your legs to the floor, keeping them straight and your toes pulled up in the direction of your face. *Do this movement very slowly once a day.*

Sitting Stretch Sit straight on the floor with your legs spread wide apart. Put the hands on the left leg just below the knee. Bend forward as far as you can, feeling the stretch on your leg. Then with short movements inch the face closer to the floor. Keep telling yourself to relax the back of your neck and shoulders as you do these short movements. Don't bounce up and down. Just use short movements *25 to 50 times*. You will feel yourself stretching and relaxing as you get closer and closer to the floor. Then switch sides and do the same thing with the other side. When you can go all the way to the floor with your abdomen against your leg, you will be stretched.

There you have them. The above exercises shouldn't take more than 10 minutes. If you are overweight, have back problems, or other physical disorders, be sure to consult your physician before attempting any of them.

POSTURE PERFECT

If you want to be kind to your body and feel good, it is essential to develop the habit of good posture, standing and sitting. Good posture permits the body to use the least amount of energy to maintain balance. It is especially important to sit with good posture. Slouching or reaching out at your desk is detrimental to your health, inhibiting digestion, circulation, and breathing. It also strains the natural spinal curves, muscles, joints, and eyes. Sitting with your elbow on the table, your head resting on your hand, inhibits body and head movement, as does slouching down in your chair.

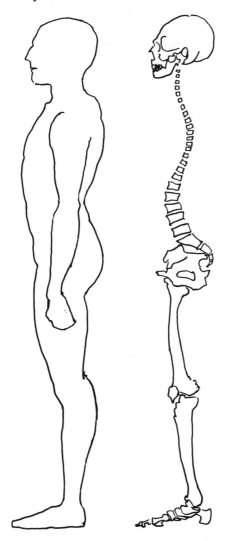

Check your posture. Standing and sitting straight means maintaining the three natural curves of your spine—the cervical (neck), thoracic (upper back), and lumbar (lower back). You will be most comfortable when you learn to use the following comfort suggestions presented on the next page.

POSTURE COMFORT SUGGESTIONS

1. Pretend that there are two balloons attached by strings to each ear and one balloon attached to the center of your chest pulling you straight up. This will automatically align your back into the correct up and down position, and the curves of your spine will be correct.

2. Keep your shoulders relaxed. Do not raise them to accommodate arm rests on your chair or to prop yourself forward or backward.

3. Make sure that your chair height is adjusted so that your feet can rest comfortably on the floor. The front of the chair seat must not press on your upper legs, causing poor circulation. If the chair seat is too high, either adjust it down or get a foot rest.

4. The top of your screen is to be even with your forehead.

5. Keep your weight slightly forward on the seat of your chair. You may want a small wedge pad placed on the back of your chair seat to help you do this.

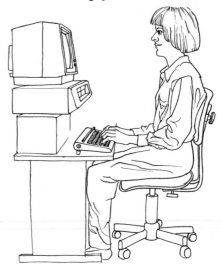

6. Hold your arms and hands at keyboard level.

7. Make sure that your eyes are at least 24″ from the surface of your screen.

8. Sit on a chair that allows free movement.

If you are not now observing the suggestions above, begin today. It takes time to change any habit, but with attention, intention, and practice, you can replace old habits with new ones and in a very short time feel much more comfortable at your work station all day long. Maintain perfect posture when you are driving, walking, watching television, and sitting on airplanes or buses. You will spare yourself discomfort, pain, and time off from work.

MASSAGE

Sore and tight muscles deserve care. When we push ourselves, sit the wrong way, become overtired, or simply work too long without a break, we can end up with knots and other soreness in our muscles. Most of the following therapies for muscle fatigue can be performed during a mini-break. They take only seconds and can make you feel wonderful.

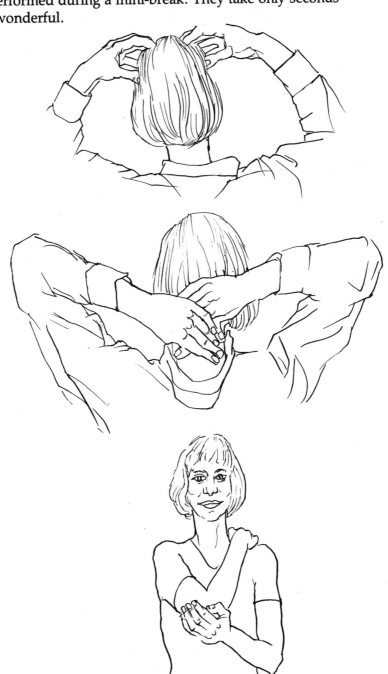

Head Beginning with the top of the head, massage your scalp with the fingers of both hands.

Neck Work down the back of your neck, squeezing the neck muscles between the thumb and forefingers of both hands.

One-Handed Massage of Neck and Shoulders With the right arm reaching across your chest and the left hand supporting the right elbow, massage the left shoulder, working up the side and the back of the neck. Then reverse hands and massage the right side.

MASSAGE (Continued)

Fingers, Hand, Arm, and Shoulder Massage With one hand, massage the other. Begin with the fingers. With your right hand, squeeze the fingers with your thumb and fingers of your left hand. Begin with the nails. Squeeze for the count of four, release, and then work your massage down the fingers to the hand. Massage the hand and then continue up the wrist, forearm upper arm, and shoulder. Work the shoulder muscles right up to your neck. People who have desk jobs often have sore shoulder muscles. Then massage the right hand, arm, and shoulder with the left hand. Always begin with the extremity and work toward your heart.

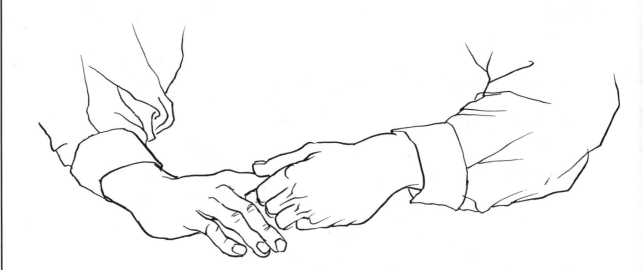

Pressure Release As you do the above, you may find places where your muscles are knotted or sore. Apply strong pressure to these areas with your thumb or finger. Continue the pressure until you feel the muscle relax. At first it may hurt, but within seconds you will feel the muscle let go and the tightness melt like butter.

Other Options If you have a friend whom you feel comfortable with, ask him or her to assist you with the hard-to-reach places on your upper back. It is also a good idea to visit a good chiropractor and/or massage therapist if you are in pain.

EATING AND DRINKING

Healthy Eating   The quantity of food we put into our bodies affects our energy level. Even though food is one of our body's energy sources, the body has to work to digest food. The more we eat, the harder it must work. For each of us there is an optimum intake that provides us with the energy we need. Eating more food than we need doesn't mean more energy; it probably means less energy to think and produce on the job. Eating more calories than we need can make us fat. Carrying around extra weight is added stress to the body. Since diet is an important part of our daily energy level, what kinds of foods we eat makes a difference. Some "foods" are not food at all but simply "taste pleasers." Many taste pleasers—sugar desserts, sugar drinks, candy, caffeine drinks—will upset your metabolism. If you have the vending machine habit, watch out. Candy bars and other packaged foods may give you a brief burst of energy, but soon you will feel tired and fatigued. Candy fools your body into thinking it has been fed, and the energy lasts only for a few minutes. Instead of candy, keep some fresh fruit in your desk drawer or in your car and eat it instead. There are many opinions on the best way to feed your body.

Liquids   People who work at workstations need to drink plenty of liquids. Companies that use computer terminals must keep interior spaces cool and dry. Such an atmosphere can cause dehydration. Symptoms of dehydration are dry eyes, dry skin, burning eyes, and thirst. It is important to drink plenty of liquids if you work in this kind of environment.

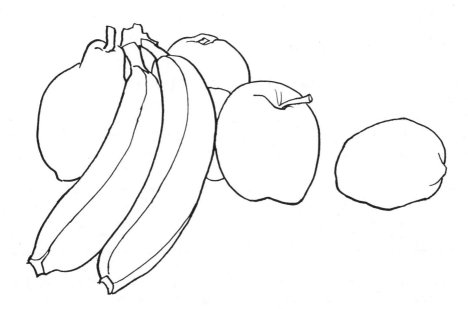

DIET AND FOOD RECOMMENDATIONS

1. Eat nutritious food—food with all the natural vitamins and minerals.

2. Eat clean food—food that is organically grown, has no preservatives, and has not been irradiated.

3. Eat fresh food—food that is in a natural state: uncooked raw fruits, vegetables, sprouts, nuts, and seeds, for example.

4. Eat only when you are hungry.

5. Never overeat and overload the stomach.

6. To insure efficient digestion, never drink coffee, tea, or water with a meal—these liquids dilute the digestive juices—slowing the digestive process. Food passes into the intestine and cannot be assimilated by the body, which equals useless eating.

7. Drink liquids between meals, especially uncooked fruit and vegetable juices.

8. Be careful how you combine your foods. Don't eat fruit with vegetables, etc. More and more research confirms that proper food combining is important for efficient digestion, because the enzymes that digest one kind of food do not digest the other.

9. Watch your cholesterol intake.

10. Remember that the best eating habits are nutritious food combinations in moderation.

Caffeine   It is very easy to get dependent on caffeine to get you through the day. And caffeine is addicting. Just because your company furnishes you with free coffee doesn't mean you must drink it. When you eat, sleep, exercise, and follow the other suggestions in this book, you won't need caffeine. You will feel vigorous and strong. You will be more productive than you ever thought possible. Instead of drinking coffee or caffeine teas, drink fruit juice, vegetable juices, and herb teas.

Plan One Week   Earlier in this book you kept a log of what you ate and drank for one week. Now, plan an ideal week. Use the chart on the next page to decide what you will eat for one week. Fill it out and follow it. See if it doesn't make a big difference in the way you feel.

	BEFORE BREAKFAST	BREAKFAST	BETWEEN BREAKFAST & LUNCH	LUNCH	BETWEEN LUNCH & DINNER	DINNER	BETWEEN DINNER & SLEEP
Monday							
Tuesday							
Wednesday							
Thursday							
Friday							
Saturday							
Sunday							

THE HURRY HABIT

This chapter could be called "The Hurry-Worry Habit." Worry and fear cause you to feel you need to hurry. Fears and beliefs that make you worry include:

1. The fear that you will be late.

2. The belief that if you move faster, you will be able to get more done.

3. The belief that if you hurry, you can arrive on time.

4. The fear that you won't finish on time.

5. The belief that you are behind and that you must catch up.

6. The fear that you will lose your job unless you are more productive.

7. The belief that you are in competition and that hurrying will give you an edge.

The hurry habit is destructive in both short-term and lifetime situations. Long-term goals necessarily reflect our short-term concerns and day-by-day activities. Impatience for success can lead to hurrying all work and recreational activities—eating, driving, walking, talking, working, exercising, loving, reading, even "having fun." We use expressions such as "It's a waste of time" and "I don't have time." People with the hurry/worry habit are usually Type A, high pressured, coronary-prone personality types who drive themselves to be productive during leisure as well as work. They sabotage their bodies by never really letting go, never giving themselves time to relax. If you commute to work, you may see these types racing down the freeway at 80 miles per hour, all the while talking on their car phones or listening to motivational tapes to help them "cope" under pressure. People who operate this way really need some more "down time."

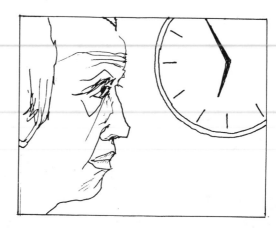

All time stress is self-inflicted. If we experience time stress, it is our own creation. Our beliefs, thinking, goals, commitments, motivations, fears, and worries make us feel "behind" and that we must rush.

If you have the hurry-worry habit, learn how to create "easy time"—time when it doesn't matter what you do. If you like, simply do nothing at all. Easy time is self-renewing, restoring physical and psychological energy. Giving yourself permission to forget pressures and play with your kids, fool around, sit, sleep, relax, listen to music, laugh, take a walk, create some form of art—draw, paint, dance, sing, play a musical instrument, or meditate—will not only be enjoyable but will leave you feeling revitalized and refreshed.

High productivity demands that we lead lives in which stress is a factor in achievement and success. The following suggestions will help you banish the hurry habit:

1. Balance stressed times with easy times.

2. Learn to disengage. Stop, take a break, relax, rest, or meditate.

3. Enjoy the experience of being alive.

4. Learn to "let go" with your body, even when you are in a stressed situation.

5. Breathe correctly while working, driving, and relaxing.

6. Read a book on time-stress management to help you effect your changes.

7. Learn to create "easy time" in your life.

THE MINI-BREAK

Any sustained activity, no matter how enjoyable, eventually becomes stressful. If you enjoy your work, that is great. But work will be even more enjoyable if you take mini-breaks every half hour. A mini-break is 30 seconds of time when you look away from your work, relax, and "let go." During this brief time, you can engage in one or more of the following:

1. Look into the distance as far as you can see.

2. Do one or two sequences of deep breathing. Relax and let go.

3. Do one or two movement exercises.

4. Do a stretching exercise.

5. Palm and deep breathe for 30 seconds.

6. Give yourself a personal message.

Below outline your schedule for mini-breaks. Enter the time and the activity for each mini-break during your typical day.

Mini-Break Schedule:

TIME   **MINI-BREAK ACTIVITY**

_____   _____

_____   _____

_____   _____

_____   _____

_____   _____

_____   _____

_____   _____

_____   _____

PSYCHOLOGICAL PRESSURE

Management Pressures   When VDT workers were interviewed, all mentioned one factor as most important. They all felt the freedom to work without being watched over and monitored every minute to be of utmost importance. Being able to get up and walk to the bathroom, get a drink, or just stand and stretch when they felt like it made the workplace much more stress free. They agreed that an environment of trust, where management allows workers to take responsibility for their jobs and and trusts them to do their best, conducive to a relaxed atmosphere and, in the end, more productive. In this kind of workplace, workers have less absenteeism and fewer health problems. Workers looked forward to going to work rather than resenting their jobs and their bosses.

A worker who is closely monitored feels intimidated and bullied. Work does not have to seem like drudgery but can be a source of pride and raise a person's sense of self-esteem. Workers are entitled to safe, healthy, relaxed environments. Workers benefit and so do their employers.

Personal Pressures   Other kinds of psychological pressure workers create for themselves. These kinds of stresses are very common and are addressed in depth in some other Crisp Publications such as: *Preventing Job Burnout, Successful Self-Management,* and *Mental Fitness*. These titles will help workers address their personal problems that can interfere with work performance. These titles can be ordered using the form in the back of this book.

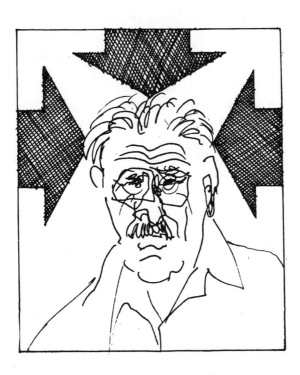

SLEEP

Sleep revitalizes our bodies and rests the eyes. We have all experienced how tired we feel after only one sleepless night. Sleep helps us to be top performers mentally and physically each day. If you want to up your productivity to work at your best, be sure that you get enough sleep and good quality sleep.

Quality Sleep Quality sleep is enough undisturbed, restful, unstressed, peaceful sleep to completely rejuvenate your body. To insure good quality sleep, you may want to do some stretching exercises just before bed to relax your muscles. The best quality sleep will be gained by going to bed early and sleeping in the dark until you awake naturally. The old adage, ''Early to bed, early to rise, makes a man healthy, wealthy, and wise,'' is good advice. The more hours we sleep before midnight the better. Go to bed early and don't eat anything at least two hours before you retire for the night.

Caffeine and Sleeping Pills If you are now dependent on sleep-inducing drugs, seek professional advice to eliminate them. Residues of these drugs in your system can cause drowsiness and dull thinking on the job. Then, you're more likely to turn to caffeine drinks—coffee, tea, or colas containing caffeine—or sugar snacks to pep you up and keep you awake during the day. Before you know it, you are drinking three, five, 10 cups of coffee and by bedtime you are still wired. Then you take your sleep-inducing drug and repeat the entire cycle the next day. This is very hard on your body.

Alcoholic Nightcaps Alcoholic nightcaps are also a bad idea. Alcohol is a depressant, and your body has to work to metabolize the alcohol while you are asleep. Often, that means a trip to the bathroom during the night, which further disturbs your sleep cycle.

Nicotine Nicotine, a central nervous system stimulant, should be discontinued well before bedtime. (Of course, smoking poses many risks to your health.) If all such substances as cigarettes, coffee, alcoholic beverages, chocolate, soft drinks, etc., are eliminated, you will notice a dramatic improvement in the quality of your sleep and your energy level. Simply avoiding them after six o'clock in the evening will make for a considerable improvement in your sleep each night.

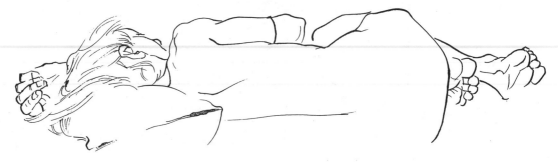

Have a Routine   Good quality sleep means not simply a sufficient length of sleep but regular, relaxed, and peaceful sleep. To achieve good quality sleep, keep your schedule regular. Eat regular meals, and go to sleep at the same time each night and rise at the same time each morning; sleeping in on weekends can upset your natural body rhythm and sleep cycles. Rising each morning at the same time no matter when you went to bed the previous night is better than trying to sleep the same number of hours each night. Your body has natural rhythms of waking, dreaming, and deep sleeping. Put the day's problems behind you. Read something enjoyable, watch some comedy on T.V., listen to music. Put yourself in a relaxed frame of mind. Forgive and forget your daytime problems. Feel at peace with yourself and the world. Do some deep breathing and relax completely.

Naps   When you are under stress, you will probably require more sleep than usual. It is better to give yourself additional rest during the day by taking a nap or meditating. Many cultures enjoy a nap after lunch and then return to work at 3:30 PM and work to 8:00 PM. Our culture does not permit this, but a 20-minute, eyes-closed rest period during the lunch hour can be very beneficial.

Sleeping Posture   Correct sleeping posture promotes good quality sleep. Treat yourself to a firm mattress. Sagging mattresses and improperly filled water beds do not provide even support to your head, neck, shoulders, spine, and hips.

Sleep on your side with your knees bent. Sometimes called the fetal position, this is the ideal sleeping position for most people. Keep both legs bent about equally. If it is uncomfortable to have your knees together, place a small pillow or pad between them. One leg dropped over the other will rotate your pelvis and twist your lower spine; avoid this position. Support your head and neck to keep your neck vertebrae and spine in alignment.

If you must sleep on your back, place a large pillow under your knees. A small pillow or a rolled up towel under your neck will help support the natural curve of your neck vertebrae.

Sleeping with your arms above your head can cause numbness and tingling in your arms and hands, pinching neck vertebrae and cramping muscles, ligaments, blood vessels, and neck and shoulder nerves.

Sleeping on your stomach causes your spine to bend, twists your head, and stresses neck muscles, ligaments, and nerves. This strain on your neck, back, spine, muscles, and nerves can cause backaches, headaches, and dull nerve pain.

Check your sleeping posture. If you have been having chronic back pain or discomfort during the day, it could be due to your sleeping posture. After all, seven or eight hours in the wrong position is a considerable amount of time to spend twisted or strained!

SLEEP (Continued)

Your Sleep Cycle   A normal sleep cycle lasts about 90 minutes. It includes light sleep, deep sleep, and rapid eye movement (REM) sleep—the dream state. Allow your body to pass through each full cycle. It is better not to depend on an alarm to wake you. Alarms alarm you! They startle you, bringing you out of sleep before you are ready. Rather, allow yourself to wake naturally. If you have to get up at a certain time, it is better to give yourself a positive suggestion upon retiring the night before. Tell yourself that you want to awake naturally at a given time. With practice, you will wake up on the minute every time. If you wish, set the alarm for five or 10 minutes after your desired waking-up time as a back-up. Soon, you will find that you can awake at your desired time without an alarm. Your body will adjust its sleep cycle, and you will feel great. Commit yourself to a regular sleep time below:

My Bed Time Routine

My regular bed time is: _____

My waking time is: _____

This is the routine that I follow each night before going to bed.

1. _____

2. _____

3. _____

4. _____

5. _____

6. _____

7. _____

8. _____

Review your bedtime routine in light of what you've just read. If any part of it doesn't make good sense, modify your habits in the interest of promoting quality sleep.

PART IV

VISION CARE

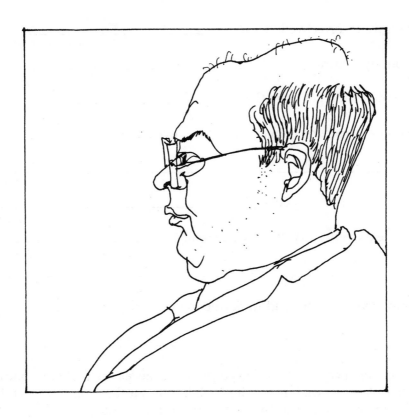

YOUR EYES: A BAROMETER OF BODY HEALTH

The health of your eyes is a barometer of your body health. If you have perfect eyesight, your vision is clear, and your eyes feel good, chances are that your body is doing well also. Do you experience any of the following symptoms? If so, describe the symptom, when it occurs, and how often you experience it.

Do you wear corrective lenses? _____

Do your eyes hurt? _____

Does your vision get blurry? _____

Do you have reccurring headaches from eye strain? _____

_____

Do you have trouble focusing? _____

Do you experience dry or burning eyes? _____

_____

Do you have a chronic stiff neck due to eye strain?_____

_____

If you experience any of these symptoms, chances are that your body is hurting in other places as well. If not, it is still important that you pay attention to this section to keep your eyes in good shape and promote good vision.

Your eyes work best when they are comfortable and relaxed. Sitting in front of a VDT is not good for your vision. The terminal is located at a fixed distance and doesn't move. Our eyes were designed to watch movement in the distance. Using them to watch a screen up close is the opposite of their designed purpose. Yet your body and eyes are very adaptable. If you are conscientious and care for your eyes, you can keep them strong in spite of the difficult tasks you are giving them.

The next section of this book deals specifically with your vision and its care. We will learn the basics of eye functioning, the mental and physical aspects of vision, and habits and exercises that can keep your eyes strong and your vision clear. If you adopt these good vision habits, you can maintain and, in some cases, even regain your good vision.

HOW YOUR EYES WORK

Light   Since we are discussing vision, it is important that we understand how the eyes work. Our eyes depend upon light to see. When there is no light, our eyes can do little. So light—its quality, brightness and location—are essential for good vision. When we look at a VDT we see organized patterns of light and dark.

Parts of the Eye   The main parts of the eye are the cornea, iris, pupil, lens, vitreous body (a jelly-like substance that fills the eye), retina (consisting of both rods and cones), the fovea centralis, and the optic nerve. See the diagram below. The shape and movement of each eye is maintained by six strong muscles. These extraocular muscles can change the shape of the eye, move it, and focus it with lightning speed. Your ability to direct both your eyes so that they focus on the same point in space is truly remarkable. The iris opens and closes the pupil, to let in more or less light. Ciliary muscles attached to the lens can change the shape of the lens to accommodate near or far vision.

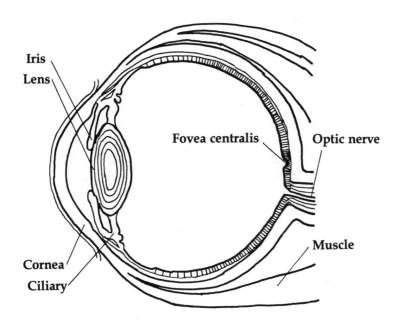

The Mental Factor   In order for you to see, light must travel through your lens and project an upside down image onto your retina. In the center of that image is the *fovea centralis,* a point on the retina where 95 percent of all the cones are located. The cones are what give us clear, colorful eyesight. The optic nerve conveys the image to the brain, where it is translated to a right-side-up recognizable image. The brain, in fact, is running the whole program called vision. According to William H. Bates, M.D., a pioneer researcher of vision improvement, ''We see very largely with the mind, and only partly with the eyes...vision depends on the mind's interpretation of the impression on the retina. What we see is not that (retinal) impression but our own impression of it.''

HOW YOUR EYES WORK (Continued)

The Saccades Muscles control the movement of the iris, the lens, and the total eye as it tracks the environment for information. Movement is the key to vision. The faster the eye moves, the better it sees. If you look closely at a friend's eye, you will notice very fast, short movements. These are called the saccades. The faster the saccades, the better your vision. When we slow down the saccades, we reduce our vision. If we stop them altogether, we see nothing. Our eye muscles control this movement. When your muscles are relaxed, the saccades move very rapidly. When your muscles are tense, the movement of the saccades slows. In Dr. Bates' opinion, "Soft, relaxed eyes see best."

The Eye Muscles The muscles that control the eye are connected to our neck muscles and our neck muscles are connected to our shoulder and upper back muscles. Therefore, if we experience tightness in these areas, it will affect our eye muscles. Stress, body tension, and immobility will cause these muscles to tighten.

Relax Your Vision Many of us tend to push our bodies and eyes to work for us. We treat them like slaves and force them to work. As you read this text, are you working to understand this information? Now, see what happens if you just allow your eyes to relax. Let your eyes blink as often as they want to, let your eyes move as fast or as slowly as they want to. When you feel like looking away, let your eyes take in the environment around you. Return to the text when your eyes feel ready. Let your eyes relax, take a deep breath, let go and read on. Performing this simple mental exercise may enable you to notice that your eyes are feeling more relaxed; your vision may even be clearer. Monitor your body and your vision during your work day. Notice how you are feeling and be aware of your state of relaxation and movement.

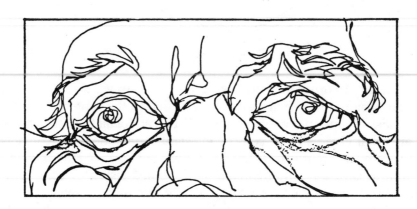

CAUSES OF EYESTRAIN AND TENSION

The Nature of the Work   Sitting at a workstation monitoring a screen, reading, studying, or reviewing written material for hours is very challenging to the lens and eye muscles. Focusing on small print and near objects for long periods of time does not exercise your full range of vision. If you make a fist and hold it tight, you will begin to feel fatigue after only a minute or two. For normal eyes to focus closely, the eye muscles need to work. People who are near-sighted have lost their natural ability to see far, usually due to long periods of time spent in close work. The muscles have changed the shape of the eyeball to be more consistent with the primary use. Eye muscles held at one distance for long periods of time, day after day, become fatigued. The eyes need frequent distant view breaks to relieve the strain.

Immobility   One of the main causes of eyestrain and tension is immobility. Sitting still for long periods of time is not healthy for the body. It is necessary for all parts of the body to continue to move all through the day. We have learned many ways to accomplish this. It is necessary for the eyes to move, too.

Staring or Spacing Out   Many of us have the habit of staring blankly into space without focusing on anything. Everything looks blurred. Some people call it daydreaming, spacing out, resting the eyes, being somewhere else for a period of time. But this habit is not restful for the eyes. The habit of staring is very common and yet very hard on the eyes. When we stare and space out we keep our eyes from moving, we slow down the saccadic eye movements. When we see someone whose eyes look aware and alive we say that their eyes sparkle. That is because the sacades are fast and lively.

Sleep   Good quality sleep revitalizes our bodies and rests the eyes. For maximum benefit to your eyes during sleep, it is recommended that you sleep in total darkness. Some people like to sleep with a light or night light on, but total black is best. Apply accupressure around your eyes. Palm your eyes for as long as possible lying in bed just before sleep and again upon waking in the morning. Do 50 swings just before retiring to relax your eyes. These four procedures will insure the maximum relaxation of the eye muscles while you sleep.

CAUSES OF EYESTRAIN
AND TENSION (Continued)

Lighting Situations   Glare and reflections on the screen, from the desk top, off walls, from stainless steel partition supports, etc., can present problems in seeing the letters, numbers, and symbols on your screen. Installing a glare filter will reduce reflections from your VDT. Locating it properly, tilting or rotating it, and having sharp resolution and good contrast on the screen can reduce eye strain.

Improperly Functioning VDT   Flickering, blur, or low contrast caused by improper functioning should be corrected immediately. Keep your machine maintained and functioning perfectly. Having sharp resolution and focus on your screen is essential to minimizing eye strain.

Eyeglasses   People who wear eyeglasses may be faced with additional problems. Wearing magnifiers, bifocals, or trifocals will mean that the head must be tilted back to focus on the screen. Neck, upper-back, shoulder problems, and headaches can result. Other reflection problems can result from glasses as well. Special computer glasses are available or a special coating can be applied to your own glasses. Consult your eye doctor for advice.

Posture   We have discussed this earlier. Constantly check your posture until you have the habit of maintaining perfect posture throughout the day. If you find that your body is too weak to sit and stand straight, do some toning exercises to strengthen the back and abdominal muscles so that you can sit and stand without slouching.

It is important that your workstation is set up to be symmetrical. The screen should be set up directly above your keys and at eye level. Workers have ended up in traction as a result of looking to the side while recording hard copy data.

Head Fixing   Head fixing is the habit of resting your head on your hand, either as a fist or using your hand as a cradle. The typical posture is to rest the elbow on the table and then prop your head up with the hand. This prevents head movement and causes immobility of the head, neck, and whole body. If you have this habit, learn to sit up with good posture. Have your fellow workers help by reminding you when you forget. Eliminate head fixing and you will eliminate one of the causes of tight necks, headaches, and eyestrain.

Squinting   When the eyes are tired, the screen is too far away, the characters on the screen are too small or blurred, and focusing becomes difficult, some people get in the habit of squinting one or both eyes. This will produce what is called the pinhole effect. You will see nearsighted people squinting for a distant sign and farsighted people squinting to read. It is a way of closing down the visual field and allowing a pinhole of light to enter the eye, therefore forcing centralization. Squinting is also common when there is too much glare. It is extremely fatiguing and in most cases will spoil normal vision for a time immediately after it is practiced. If you squint, break yourself of the habit, practice good vision habits, or wear your prescribed corrective lenses. Although wearing glasses is not encouraged unless you can't see without them, glasses are better for you than squinting.

Other Cases   Poor diet, the wrong chair, long hours, the hurry-worry habit, and lack of exercise all have a major effect on your body and eyes. These have all been discussed in other chapters.

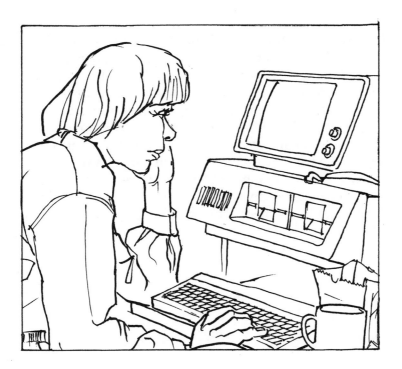

HOW TO MINIMIZE EYE STRAIN AND TENSION AT THE WORKSTATION

Drawing You can add movement to the eyes and head by introducing the "nose pencil." This is an imaginary pencil that extends from your nose to the exact point of your visual attention. As you work, you use this device to follow the words or lines on the screen in front of you—up and down or back and forth. The pencil goes wherever your interest goes. The nose pencil extends from the farthest point your eye can see to the closest point. It is totally flexible. Take your attention away from this book for a moment and view the room with your nose pencil. Find an object in the room and move your nose pencil around the contours of that object as if you were drawing the outline of the object. Now do this with two more objects. Each time, pick an object at a different distance. Notice how your head will move as you trace the object. Now do this with the words you are reading. Notice that your head now moves back and forth along the lines as you read with your nose pencil.

Most of us have the habit of holding our heads still. We were taught to do this in school. We were told that the proper way to read was to keep our heads still and let our eyes do the moving. Get in the habit of moving your head as you read, allowing your nose pencil to follow the lines.

Centralization What can drawing with the nose pencil do for you? The eye sees best at that one small point on the retina called the *fovea centralis*. Putting your sight line directly into the *fovea centralis* is called "centralization." We do this by seeing precise small details all the time, up close or in the distance. The eye does not see everything clearly. It only sees clearly at the fovea. At the fovea, vision is at least 20/20. Just 10 degrees off of the fovea, our vision is reduced to 20/400, within the realm of legal blindness. As we look around, we are constantly darting from one point to another. We do this so fast that it gives us the illusion that we see everything clearly. The nose pencil helps us to centralize on the details around us. As you pencil the environment or your work, you will be centralizing automatically moment by moment. This will also help prevent the possibility of staring or spacing out so that the saccadic eye movements stay lively and fast. Draw with your nose pencil—make it a habit!

Shifting   Another helpful habit is to shift your vision from near to far. Position yourself in your room so that you can see beyond your screen at least 20 feet. If you can see out of a window and into infinity, that is ideal. If this is not possible, a poor substitute is a poster or large photograph on the wall in front of your table. That way, you can look into the natural landscape by way of a photographic image of some pleasing scene—a beach, mountains, forests, waterfalls, etc. This shifting is good exercise for the eyes and helps them move from the fixed plane of sight—your screen. Remember to use the nose pencil when you look into the distance, just as you do on your screen.

Blinking   People who work at VDTs need to blink often. A blink every second is not too much. Some people have been taught not to blink, or that it is a sign of weakness to blink. Blinking is recommended in this program to keep your eyes rested and lubricated. The brief moment when your eyes are closed is a short rest period for the eyes. If you suffer from burning or dry eyes, you probably are not blinking enough. The air in many of the spaces that workers occupy with desk machines is characteristically dry. To offset this dryness, blink frequently and drink plenty of liquids.

Yawning   In some social circles yawning is not acceptable: however, there are arguments to have it "legalized." Yawning is a natural body function that does you a lot of good. Yawning oxygenates the blood by bringing into the head and lungs a large supply of oxygen all at once. You will also notice that yawning leaves your eyes feeling nice and moist. When we yawn, our eyes usually form tears, in the process lubricating the eyes. Janet Goodrich, who wrote the book *Natural Vision Improvement* says, "We must become champion yawners."

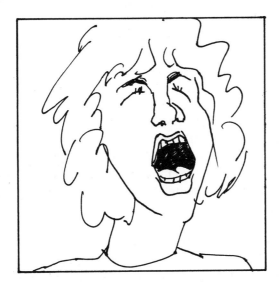

Palming Cup your hands slightly with your fingers together. Cover your eyes with your hands in this way so that they block out all the light. The hands do not press against the eyes but simply cover the closed eyes. You can palm as much as you like. Do it frequently during the day. The process is very relaxing for the eyes. If you notice that you are having difficulty focusing during long periods of work at your terminal, palm and breathe deeply for a few minutes to relax the eyes and regain your sight.

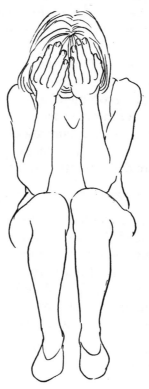

Accupressure If you visit China, you would notice that very few Chinese people wear glasses. Even the older people have good eyesight. The Chinese are taught in school how to take care of their eyes. One of the things that they learn is to practice accupressure around their eyes. The diagram on the following page shows you the accupressure points so that you can practice this on your own eyes. With both hands, press on each of these points for about six seconds and then release. Breathe, and then move to the next point. Doing this two or three times during the day will be very beneficial in keeping your eyes relaxed and your vision clear.

If you incorporate these simple practices into your day, your eyes will feel and see better. Keeping the eyes relaxed will strengthen them and minimize the possibility of vision loss or other eye disorders due to working conditions.

ACCUPRESSURE POINTS

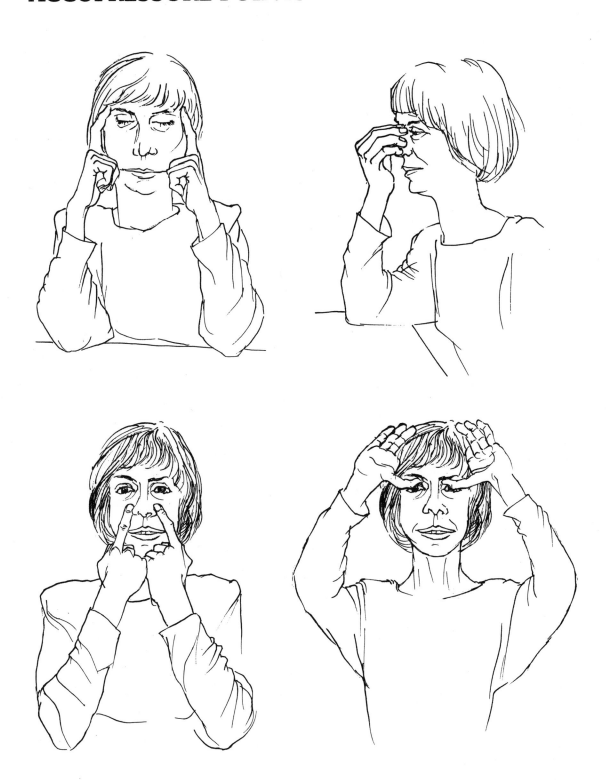

PART V

DEVELOPING A PERSONAL ACTION PLAN

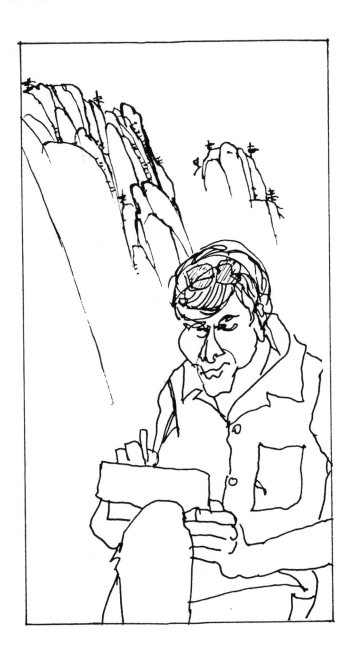

GOAL SETTING

Now that you know what to do, what are you going to do? It is time to commit to paper the program you have outlined for yourself. Write down your goals. What are you going to do to begin right now? What will your progress be in one month? And what will you have accomplished six months from now? Don't get carried away and try to do it all at once. Take it one step at a time. Prioritize your program and proceed with the most important things first.

What I am going to do this week is:

_____

_____

_____

What I am going to accomplish in the next 30 days is:

_____

_____

_____

_____

My goals for the next six months are:

_____

_____

_____

_____

_____

It is important to visualize your goals. Picture what you are going to do in your mind. Draw out what you are going to do in pictures or in words. Use the illustrations in this book or cut out pictures from magazines. Post words and images that will help you remember your goals.

RECOMMENDATIONS IN BRIEF

Here is a list of recommendations that summarize the text of this book. Use your commuting time to and from work as relaxing time.

Move a lot.

Use waiting time to breathe deeply.

Stretch your body often.

Move your head when you read anything.

When you are feeling low, talk to a friend.

Massage yourself, especially where it hurts.

Minimize your use of sugar, salt, caffeine, and alcohol.

Eat real food.

Drink and blink at work.

Connect with nature at least once a day.

Sleep on your side in peace.

Every month, take the time to look inside. Listen to your heart. Look at where you are and where you are going.

Get in the habit of letting go with your body.

Do something creative each day that gives you pleasure. It will energize you. Play, sing, or hum a tune, draw or paint a picture, write a poem, work in your garden.

Exercise daily.

Do one thing at a time.

Work with focus and intention.

See with soft relaxed eyes.

Sit and stand tall. Teach yourself the habit of good posture.

Prioritize your daily activities.

Take mini-breaks during your day.

Learn to laugh at yourself and life.

Listen and forgive.

SUGGESTED READINGS

Bates, Williams H. *Better Eyesight Without Glasses.* New York, NY: Henry Holt and Company, 1968.

Corbett, Margaret Darst. *Help Yourself To Better Sight.* Englewood Cliffs, NJ: Prentice-Hall, Inc., 1949.

Dennison, Paul. *Switching On.* Glendale, CA: Edu-Kinesthetics, Inc., 1981.

Diamond, Harvey and Marilyn. *Fit For Life II: Living Health.* New York, NY: Warner Books, 1987, Revised 1989.

Donkin, Scott W., D. C. *Sitting on the Job.* Boston, MA: Houghton Mifflin Company, 1989.

Fonda, Jane. *Jane Fonda's Workout Book.* New York, NY: Simon and Schuster, 1981.

Goodrich, Janet, Ph.D. *Natural Vision Improvement.* Berkeley, CA: Celestial Arts, 1985.

Huxley, Aldous. *The Art Of Seeing.* Seattle, WA: Montana Books, 1975.

Pinckney, Callan. *Callanetics: 10 Years Younger in 10 Hours.* New York, NY: William Morrow and Company, Inc., 1984.

Pulgram, William L., A.I.A. and Stones, Richard. *Designing the Automated Office.* New York, NY: Watson-Guptill Publications, 1984.

Schneider, Meir. *Self Healing My Life and Vision.* New York, NY and London, England: Routledge & Kegan, Paul, 1987.

Selby, John. *The Visual Handbook.* Shaftesbury, Dorest, England: Element Books, 1987.

NOTES

FOR OTHER FIFTY-MINUTE SELF-STUDY BOOKS
SEE ORDER FORM AT THE BACK OF THE BOOK.

NOTES

THE FIFTY-MINUTE SERIES

Quantity	Title	Code #	Price	Amount
	MANAGEMENT TRAINING			
	Self-Managing Teams	000-0	$7.95	
	Delegating For Results	008-6	$7.95	
	Successful Negotiation—Revised	09-2	$7.95	
	Increasing Employee Productivity	010-8	$7.95	
	Personal Performance Contracts—Revised	12-2	$7.95	
	Team Building—Revised	16-5	$7.95	
	Effective Meeting Skills	33-5	$7.95	
	An Honest Day's Work: Motivating Employees To Excel	39-4	$7.95	
	Managing Disagreement Constructively	41-6	$7.95	
	Training Managers To Train	43-2	$7.95	
	Learning To Lead	043-4	$7.95	
	The Fifty-Minute Supervisor—Revised	58-0	$7.95	
	Leadership Skills For Women	62-9	$7.95	
	Systematic Problem Solving & Decision Making	63-7	$7.95	
	Coaching & Counseling	68-8	$7.95	
	Ethics In Business	69-6	$7.95	
	Understanding Organizational Change	71-8	$7.95	
	Project Management	75-0	$7.95	
	Risk Taking	76-9	$7.95	
	Managing Organizational Change	80-7	$7.95	
	Working Together In A Multi-Cultural Organization	85-8	$7.95	
	Selecting And Working With Consultants	87-4	$7.95	
	PERSONNEL MANAGEMENT			
	Your First Thirty Days: A Professional Image in a New Job	003-5	$7.95	
	Office Management: A Guide To Productivity	005-1	$7.95	
	Men and Women: Partners at Work	009-4	$7.95	
	Effective Performance Appraisals—Revised	11-4	$7.95	
	Quality Interviewing—Revised	13-0	$7.95	
	Personal Counseling	14-9	$7.95	
	Attacking Absenteeism	042-6	$7.95	
	New Employee Orientation	46-7	$7.95	
	Professional Excellence For Secretaries	52-1	$7.95	
	Guide To Affirmative Action	54-8	$7.95	
	Writing A Human Resources Manual	70-X	$7.95	
	Winning at Human Relations	86-6	$7.95	
	WELLNESS			
	Mental Fitness	15-7	$7.95	
	Wellness in the Workplace	020-5	$7.95	
	Personal Wellness	021-3	$7.95	

THE FIFTY-MINUTE SERIES (Continued)

Quantity	Title	Code #	Price	Amount
	WELLNESS (CONTINUED)			
	Preventing Job Burnout	23-8	$7.95	
	Job Performance and Chemical Dependency	27-0	$7.95	
	Overcoming Anxiety	029-9	$7.95	
	Productivity at the Workstation	041-8	$7.95	
	COMMUNICATIONS			
	Technical Writing In The Corporate World	004-3	$7.95	
	Giving and Receiving Criticism	023-X	$7.95	
	Effective Presentation Skills	24-6	$7.95	
	Better Business Writing—Revised	25-4	$7.95	
	Business Etiquette And Professionalism	032-9	$7.95	
	The Business Of Listening	34-3	$7.95	
	Writing Fitness	35-1	$7.95	
	The Art Of Communicating	45-9	$7.95	
	Technical Presentation Skills	55-6	$7.95	
	Making Humor Work	61-0	$7.95	
	Visual Aids In Business	77-7	$7.95	
	Speed-Reading In Business	78-5	$7.95	
	Publicity Power	82-3	$7.95	
	Influencing Others	84-X	$7.95	
	SELF-MANAGEMENT			
	Attitude: Your Most Priceless Possession-Revised	011-6	$7.95	
	Personal Time Management	22-X	$7.95	
	Successful Self-Management	26-2	$7.95	
	Balancing Home And Career—Revised	035-3	$7.95	
	Developing Positive Assertiveness	38-6	$7.95	
	The Telephone And Time Management	53-X	$7.95	
	Memory Skills In Business	56-4	$7.95	
	Developing Self-Esteem	66-1	$7.95	
	Creativity In Business	67-X	$7.95	
	Managing Personal Change	74-2	$7.95	
	Stop Procrastinating: Get To Work!	88-2	$7.95	
	CUSTOMER SERVICE/SALES TRAINING			
	Sales Training Basics—Revised	02-5	$7.95	
	Restaurant Server's Guide—Revised	08-4	$7.95	
	Telephone Courtesy And Customer Service	18-1	$7.95	
	Effective Sales Management	031-0	$7.95	
	Professional Selling	42-4	$7.95	
	Customer Satisfaction	57-2	$7.95	
	Telemarketing Basics	60-2	$7.95	
	Calming Upset Customers	65-3	$7.95	
	Quality At Work	72-6	$7.95	
	Managing Quality Customer Service	83-1	$7.95	
	Quality Customer Service—Revised	95-5	$7.95	
	SMALL BUSINESS AND FINANCIAL PLANNING			
	Understanding Financial Statements	022-1	$7.95	
	Marketing Your Consulting Or Professional Services	40-8	$7.95	

THE FIFTY-MINUTE SERIES (Continued)

Quantity	Title	Code #	Price	Amount
	SMALL BUSINESS AND FINANCIAL PLANNING (CONTINUED)			
	Starting Your New Business	44-0	$7.95	
	Personal Financial Fitness—Revised	89-0	$7.95	
	Financial Planning With Employee Benefits	90-4	$7.95	
	BASIC LEARNING SKILLS			
	Returning To Learning: Getting Your G.E.D.	002-7	$7.95	
	Study Skills Strategies—Revised	05-X	$7.95	
	The College Experience	007-8	$7.95	
	Basic Business Math	024-8	$7.95	
	Becoming An Effective Tutor	028-0	$7.95	
	CAREER PLANNING			
	Career Discovery	07-6	$7.95	
	Effective Networking	030-2	$7.95	
	Preparing for Your Interview	033-7	$7.95	
	Plan B: Protecting Your Career	48-3	$7.95	
	I Got the Job!	59-9	$7.95	
	RETIREMENT			
	Personal Financial Fitness—Revised	89-0	$7.95	
	Financial Planning With Employee Benefits	90-4	$7.95	

OTHER CRISP INC. BOOKS

Quantity	Title	Code #	Price	Amount
	Desktop Publishing	001-9	$ 5.95	
	Stepping Up To Supervisor	11-8	$13.95	
	The Unfinished Business Of Living: Helping Aging Parents	19-X	$12.95	
	Managing Performance	23-7	$19.95	
	Be True To Your Future: A Guide To Life Planning	47-5	$13.95	
	Up Your Productivity	49-1	$10.95	
	Comfort Zones: Planning Your Future 2/e	73-4	$13.95	
	Copyediting 2/e	94-7	$18.95	
	Recharge Your Career	027-2	$12.95	
	Practical Time Management	275-4	$13.95	

VIDEO TITLE*

Quantity	Video Title*	Code #	Preview	Purchase	Amount
	Attitude: Your Most Priceless Possession	012-4	$25.00	$395.00	
	Quality Customer Service	013-2	$25.00	$395.00	
	Team Building	014-2	$25.00	$395.00	
	Job Performance & Chemical Dependency	015-9	$25.00	$395.00	
	Better Business Writing	016-7	$25.00	$395.00	
	Comfort Zones	025-6	$25.00	$395.00	
	Creativity in Business	036-1	$25.00	$395.00	
	Motivating at Work	037-X	$25.00	$395.00	
	Calming Upset Customers	040-X	$25.00	$395.00	
	Balancing Home and Career	048-5	$25.00	$395.00	
	Stress and Mental Fitness	049-3	$25.00	$395.00	

(*Note: All tapes are VHS format. Video package includes five books and a Leader's Guide.)

THE FIFTY-MINUTE SERIES
(Continued)

	Amount
Total Books	
Less Discount (5 or more different books 20% sampler)	
Total Videos	
Less Discount (purchase of 3 or more videos earn 20%)	
Shipping ($3.50 per video, $.50 per book)	
California Tax (California residents add 7%)	
TOTAL	

☐ Send volume discount information.

☐ Please send me a catalog.

☐ Mastercard ☐ VISA ☐ AMEX

Exp. Date _____

Account No. _____ Name (as appears on card) _____

Ship to: _____ Bill to: _____

_____ _____

_____ _____

_____ _____

Phone number: _____ P.O. # _____

All orders except those with a P.O.# must be prepaid.
For more information Call (415) 949-4888 or FAX (415) 949-1610.

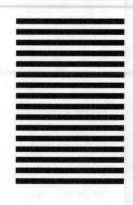

NO POSTAGE
NECESSARY
IF MAILED
IN THE
UNITED STATES

BUSINESS REPLY
FIRST CLASS   PERMIT NO. 884   LOS ALTOS, CA

POSTAGE WILL BE PAID BY ADDRESSEE

Crisp Publications, Inc.
95 First Street
Los Altos, CA 94022